MW01286132

TREATING RISKY AND COMPULSIVE BEHAVIOR IN TRAUMA SURVIVORS

Treating Risky and Compulsive Behavior in Trauma Survivors

John Briere

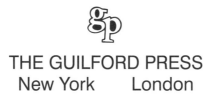

THE GUILFORD PRESS
New York   London

The author has checked with sources believed to be reliable in his efforts to provide
information that is complete and generally in accord with the standards of practice that
are accepted at the time of publication. However, in view of the possibility of human error
or changes in behavioral, mental health, or medical sciences, neither the author, nor
the editor and publisher, nor any other party who has been involved in the preparation
or publication of this work warrants that the information contained herein is in every
respect accurate or complete, and they are not responsible for any errors or omissions
or the results obtained from the use of such information. Readers are encouraged to
confirm the information contained in this book with other sources.

Library of Congress Cataloging-in-Publication Data

Names: Briere, John, author.
Title: Treating risky and compulsive behavior in trauma survivors / John Briere.
Description: New York : The Guilford Press, [2019] | Includes bibliographical references
    and index.
Identifiers: LCCN 2018053923 | ISBN 9781462538683 (hardback : alk. paper)
Subjects: | MESH: Self-Injurious Behavior—therapy | Adult Survivors of Child
    Adverse Events—psychology | Dangerous Behavior | Psychological Trauma—therapy |
    Psychotherapy—methods
Classification: LCC RC569.5.S48 | NLM WM 165 | DDC 616.85/820651—dc23
LC record available at https://lccn.loc.gov/2018053923

About the Author

John Briere, PhD, is Professor of Psychiatry and Behavioral Sciences at the Keck School of Medicine, University of Southern California (USC); Director of the USC Adolescent Trauma Training Center of the National Child Traumatic Stress Network; and Remote Program Faculty at the Institute for Meditation and Psychotherapy. Past president of the International Society for Traumatic Stress Studies (ISTSS), Dr. Briere is a recipient of the Award for Outstanding Contributions to the Science of Trauma Psychology from Division 56 of the American Psychological Association and the Robert S. Laufer Memorial Award for Scientific Achievement from ISTSS, among other honors. At USC, he teaches and consults in the burn center and in the inpatient psychiatry and emergency services. He lectures internationally on trauma, therapy, and mindfulness.

Acknowledgments

I would like to thank the many clinicians, researchers, trainees, and mindfulness teachers who provided helpful suggestions or input on this book, including Elaine Eaton, Diana Elliott, Barbara Gilbert, Natacha Godbout, Mandy Habib, John Jimenez, Gill Morton, Caroline Newton, Lori Queen, Marsha Runtz, Catherine Scott, Randye Semple, Beth Sternleib, and Sarah Stoycos. Special thanks to Erin Eadie for her edits and suggestions on various drafts of the manuscript, Victor Labruna and Constance Dalenberg for their substantive feedback on a nearly final version, and Tara Brach for helpful discussions around self-compassion and the ReGAIN exercise. Much appreciation to Kitty Moore, Executive Editor at The Guilford Press, for her interest in my work over the years and for her insightful ideas for this book. Wonderful that we finally landed on this project! Appreciation also to Anna Nelson, Senior Production Editor at Guilford, for her able assistance. Special thanks to Bruce and Jean Lanktree for sharing their cottage—and stimulating conversations—on Georgian Bay, where significant parts of this book were written. As always, I am deeply indebted to Cheryl Lanktree for decades of love and support, and for her line-by-line reviews of this and previous books.

Contents

Introduction

It is Wednesday, 3:25 P.M. and your client, Alicia, is late.[1] This is concerning for several reasons. It has been 2 months since she last overdosed on pills and alcohol, and she is still in the rocky, on-again, off-again relationship that triggered that emergency room visit. As worrisome, her self-cutting behavior is back. And there were several hang-up calls on your voice mail this morning. It could have been from her, but you are not sure. Was she trying to reach out? Is she OK? Is she back in the hospital? Or worse?

You have been treating Alicia for over a year. She has been through much, with many ups and downs, but you are impressed and touched by her tenacity and willingness to stay in therapy despite what it brings up for her. You know that connection is hard; her childhood was filled with violence, sexual abuse, and very little love, and she battles with fear, need, and emptiness—with you, with her partner, and, for that matter, with the rest of her world. In her desperation, Alicia does things that are obviously self-harmful. She self-injures, binge drinks, sometimes attempts suicide, and is episodically unfaithful to her partner, even though her relationship with that person is one of the most important things in her life.

There is no simple guidance for the clinician at times like this. Being a psychotherapist almost invariably means working with traumatized people, some of whom endanger themselves in one way or another. Those who have been hurt in childhood, whether through abuse, neglect, invalidating environments, or insecure attachment, are at significant risk for

---

[1] All case examples presented in this book, including names and demographics, are fictional in their current form and are compiled from the stories and statements of multiple individuals.

self-injury, suicidal behavior, risky sexual activities, bingeing and purging, and a host of other seemingly impulsive, compulsive, and/or addictive activities.

Not only are such behaviors self-endangering, they also seem contradictory. Some people cut on themselves without suicidal intent, or attempt suicide but seem more in search of support or caring attention than actually wanting to die. Others pursue frequent but short-lived sexual interactions that are unfulfilling and induce shame, or repeatedly eat beyond fullness, then purge through vomiting or laxatives. Some risk serious social consequences by shoplifting inexpensive items that they do not want or need. Some hit, lie, or cheat, when what they really want is to be cared for and to care for others in return.

This makes no obvious sense. Why would a person intentionally engage in life-threatening or self-defeating activities, especially when they lead to additional emotional pain and social alienation? Freud's pleasure principle holds that humans are innately invested in pursuing pleasure and avoiding pain. If so, why do some people repeatedly do things that lead to negative outcomes rather than positive ones?

For mental health clinicians, the answer is obvious, albeit ultimately misleading: We are taught that chronically illogical behavior means psychopathology—people do these irrational things because there is something wrong with them; their behaviors are symptoms of a disorder. Once that is our conclusion, our next task is to decide which diagnosis to apply. The options are several: borderline or antisocial personality disorder? Or perhaps a conduct disorder, if the client is younger? Obsessive–compulsive disorder, or an impulse-control disorder? Maybe a behavioral addiction disorder?

Obviously, diagnosis can be part of our clinical task, and determining the proper DSM-5 (American Psychiatric Association, 2013) label for specific clinical presentations is often helpful. But diagnosis also can be recursive: We may define the disorder by referring to the behavior, and explain the behavior by referring to the diagnosis. For example, we may say that Alicia is "a borderline" because she self-injures, then explain her self-injury as being due to her borderline personality disorder. In this context, coming to a diagnostic conclusion about dysfunctional behavior may, at best, be a descriptive endeavor as opposed to an explanatory one. To say that self-injury is a borderline activity does not explain why Alicia cuts on herself, nor does it help us much to help her.

Another View

Fortunately, there is another perspective. Advances in trauma and attachment psychology suggest that many seemingly dysfunctional behaviors serve adaptive, if not homeostatic, functions, especially for those who were exposed to adversity in childhood. Based on this growing body of research, we will explore a *reactive avoidance* (RA) model that addresses activities ranging from self-injury to compulsive gambling—framing them not as manifestations of psychological illness but rather as attempts to distract, numb, block, or otherwise avoid distress associated with triggered, highly painful memories. From an RA perspective, such behaviors will be referred to as *distress reduction behaviors* (hereafter referred to as DRBs), as opposed to traditional terms such as *acting-out, dysfunctional, self-defeating*, or *impulsive* behaviors.

Although the principles of RA-focused treatment are formally introduced in this book, few of the ideas presented here are brand new. Many have been adapted from well-established treatment approaches, ranging from psychodynamic psychotherapy and interpersonal therapy to dialectical behavior therapy, mindfulness training, and exposure therapy. RA theory is also strongly influenced by several relatively new areas of research, including memory reconsolidation, inhibitory learning, suppression effects, and the limits of exposure-based habituation. These approaches and findings, in turn, are integrated with philosophies that focus on increasing self-determination, empowerment, skills development, and psychological growth, and that deemphasize pathology-based perspectives.

The RA model suggests that the goal of many so-called "maladaptive" behaviors is not self-destructiveness, but instead pain relief and, from the person's perspective, emotional survival. These activities appear illogical, because their basis is internal, and therefore largely invisible to others. And their suddenness makes them seem impulsive, when, in fact, their rapid emergence has more to do with desperation—the need to quickly reduce emotional pain before it can overwhelm limited emotional regulation skills and produce greater suffering.

A major advantage of a functional analysis of problem behaviors, in contrast to a solely diagnostic one, is that it more directly informs clinical practice. For example, if we could intervene in the actual psychological processes underlying risky sexual behavior or suicide "gestures"—whether by processing painful memories or by increasing emotional regulation capacity—we might be more effective than if we tried to treat broadly defined "borderline personality" or "conduct disorder" per se. To the extent that a functional analysis leads to specific interventions, the latter are less likely to pathologize or stigmatize, because they arise from a deconstructed perspective that views problem behaviors as reality-based, adaptive strategies, albeit ones that may require adjustment, updating, or replacement.

Notably, because the avoidance behaviors described in this book are typically side effects of unprocessed childhood trauma and early attachment problems, the treatment philosophy and methods presented here, albeit focused on reducing harmful behavior, are ultimately directed toward these broader difficulties. This means that successful intervention in a given avoidance behavior usually reflects improvement in chronic trauma- and attachment-related phenomena in general. To the extent that this occurs, other signs of heightened well-being are likely to emerge as well.

One Size Rarely Fits All

Given the complex etiologies of the behaviors described in this book, different clients may require more of certain treatment components outlined here and less of others. The need to select or modify interventions as a function of the client's background, history, and specific behaviors is not surprising. Our field is increasingly finding that the greater the complexity of what we seek to treat, the less likely one approach or technique will work for everyone, and the greater the need for case-by-case customization (Briere & Lanktree, 2012; Cloitre, 2015; Wagner, Rizvi, & Harned, 2007). For example, some clients might require even more attention to attachment-era memories and emotional regulation problems, whereas others might especially gain from processing later, explicit trauma memories and learning to manage triggered cognitive–emotional states. Some DRB-involved people initially present for treatment in mid- to older-adolescence and struggle with emergent developmental issues, whereas others seek therapy later in life, when such behaviors have become ingrained, automatic, and less directly related to childhood experiences. Certain DRBs are more prevalent in one sex than another, requiring interventions that take into account the unique social and historical experiences associated with different patterns of gender socialization.

The Sociocultural Context

Any modern treatment text, especially one focused on the effects of maltreatment, must take into account cultural differences and social inequality. Clients from different cultures, subcultures, genders, orientations, and socioeconomic backgrounds vary in their experience of—and responses to—childhood adversity (e.g., Fontes, 2005). Although many children in North American society are at risk of maltreatment, it is an unavoidable reality that institutionalized racism, sexism, homophobia and transphobia, and poverty increase the likelihood of child abuse and neglect (e.g., Arreola, Neilands, & Diaz, 2009; Klevens & Ports, 2017; Lanier, Maguire-Jack, Walsh, Drake, & Hubel, 2014), and are, themselves, broadly traumagenic (Briere, 1992; DeGruy, 2005; Pachter & Coll, 2009). This means that assessment of child maltreatment in DRB-involved individuals must not only delineate specific instances of trauma exposure but also take into account the cultural context in which such clients are living, and how social maltreatment impacts their lives at multiple levels. In this larger context, therapy also may have to address the childhood effects of social discrimination and marginalization as they affect the client's life and motivate his or her survival responses (Briere & Lanktree, 2012).

Beyond Survival

The research and clinical perspectives outlined in this book suggests an empirically informed way forward for Alicia, one that supports her in doing what she is already trying to do: survive despite a multitude of triggers, memories, and overwhelming emotions. At the same time, RA-focused therapy ultimately requires more than "just" survival. The client is also encouraged to form a therapeutic relationship, even though relationships have been dangerous in the past; to feel and process what she has spent years avoiding; and to struggle against long-held patterns of behavior that, while immediately reinforcing, ultimately increase danger and produce greater suffering. As we will see, this path is not easy or simple, but it offers Alicia the possibility of not only safety but also greater empowerment and well-being.

CHAPTER 1

Reactive Avoidance and Risky Behavior

Roshawna is a 19-year-old woman who was brought to the emergency room (ER) by paramedics following an overdose on 20 Advils and eight Imodium tablets. She reports five previous ER admissions for suicidal or self-cutting behavior, two of which were in the last month, and a history of juvenile detentions for prostitution, shoplifting, and truancy. Previous medical records indicate, variously, diagnoses of major depression, polysubstance abuse, borderline personality disorder, posttraumatic stress disorder, and bipolar disorder. Roshawna describes having been sexual abused by her father from ages 4–12 years, and chronically neglected by her mother, including having been "kicked out" of her home as a 14-year-old, with no attention to her subsequent safety or well-being. Previous admission records also describe a history of multiple sexual assaults by peers, although she currently denies any such experiences.

A review of the clinical literature reveals a number of seemingly dysfunctional or self-defeating behavior patterns, all of which are more common among those with childhood histories of abuse, neglect, and/or insecure attachment. Beyond problematic substance use and dissociation, which are considered separately, they include

- Intentional self-injury (Briere & Eadie, 2016)
- Triggered suicidal behavior (Hjelmeland & Knizek, 2010)
- Risky or compulsive sexual behavior (Vaillancourt-Morel et al., 2015)

7

- Food bingeing and purging (Rosenbaum & White, 2013)
- Compulsive gambling (American Psychiatric Association, 2013)
- Compulsive shoplifting (American Psychiatric Association, 2013)
- Reactive aggression (Fite, Raine, Stouthamer-Loeber, Loeber, & Pardini, 2009)
- Thrill- or sensation-seeking behavior (Harden, Carlson, Kretsch, Corbin, & Fromme, 2015)
- Compulsive skin picking and hair pulling (Stein et al., 2010)
- Fire setting (Blanco et al., 2010)
- Extensive preoccupation with Internet activities (Charlton & Danforth, 2007).

Given the range of these behaviors, it seems unlikely that they share similar etiologies. Yet research and clinical experience suggest that multiple types of problem behavior tend to arise from the same processes, co-occur in the same individuals, and have certain characteristics and functions in common (Briere, Hodges, & Godbout, 2010; Goodman, 2008; Grant & Chamberlain, 2014; Hayes, Wilson, Gifford, Follette, & Strosahl, 1996).

This overlap has led to several disorder-based theories concerning the development and maintenance of problematic or risky behavior. Specifically, activities such as self-injury, suicide attempts, angry outbursts, aggression, and compulsive sex, eating, or gambling have been linked in the clinical literature to one or more of three major psychiatric conditions: borderline personality disorder (BPD), impulse-control disorder, and behavioral addiction, as well as, in adolescents, conduct and oppositional defiant disorders. Although one might also include antisocial personality disorder in this list, that diagnosis focuses on less DRB-related problems, for example decreased empathy, callousness, lack of remorse, and an inflated sense of self (American Psychiatric Association, 2013)—issues that, although also potentially related to childhood adversity, generally fall outside the purview of this book.

Borderline Personality Disorder

BPD has been described as "a pervasive pattern of instability of interpersonal relationships, self-image, and affects, and marked impulsivity beginning by early adulthood and present in a variety of contexts" (American Psychiatric Association, 2000, p. 706). DSM-5 notes that BPD is characterized by episodes of disinhibition and impulsivity, during which time the client engages in risk-taking or potentially self-damaging activities, generally in response to unwanted events or triggered emotional distress, largely without consideration of personal danger.

Early descriptions of BPD stressed nonspecific "ego weakness" associated with a "borderline personality organization," in which there was significant reality distortion, immature and maladaptive defenses, and primitive or disorganized internal representations of self and others (e.g., Kernberg, 1975). Critical to classic formulations of BPD, and still present in some clinical approaches, was the idea that self-endangering behaviors reflect "acting out" of distressing unconscious material, and/or intentional manipulation to obtain nurturance, attention, or support from others (Kernberg, 1975). These behaviors were often attributed to the mother of the soon-to-be borderline's client, who was thought to punish the client's early attempts at separation and individuation, primarily by withdrawing attention and affection (Mahler, Pine, & Bergman, 1975; Masterson & Rinsley, 1975). Such deprivation was hypothesized to lead to later, often desperate, attempts to avoid abandonment in close relationships.

In contrast, recent research increasingly documents the role of child maltreatment and child–caretaker attachment disturbance—rather than maternal punishment of autonomy—in the development of BPD (e.g., Ball & Links, 2009; Godbout, Daspe, Runtz, Cyr, & Briere, 2018; Johnson, Cohen, Brown, Smailes, & Bernstein, 1999; Scott et al., 2013). The growing realization that BPD may arise, in part, from early abuse and neglect has led various clinicians and researchers to suggest that BPD may be equivalent to Herman's (1992a) *complex posttraumatic stress disorder*, a trauma syndrome that involves similar symptoms, including emotional dysregulation, easily activated childhood memories, and triggered DRBs (Cloitre, Garvert, Weiss, Carlson, & Bryant, 2014; Ford & Courtois, 2014).

Despite some similarities, however, these models are likely not equivalent (Cloitre et al., 2014), and neither (especially BPD) appears to fully explain the breadth and etiology of risky behaviors in maltreated individuals (for further discussion, see Briere & Scott, 2015; Cloitre et al., 2014; Ford & Courtois, 2014). Furthermore, the diagnosis of BPD, itself, is the subject of considerable methodological and theoretical debate (e.g., Dahl, 2008; Lewis & Grenyer, 2009; New, Triebwasser, & Charney, 2008; Paris, 2007), with some questioning whether it represents a unique disorder, or is, rather, a heterogeneous collection of symptoms and problems that overlap with other disorders—including those related to trauma and attachment disturbance (e.g., Akiskal, 2004; Briere & Rickards, 2007; Cloitre et al., 2014; Kulkarni, 2017; Paris, 2007).

Whatever the ultimate validity of BPD as an explanation for DRBs and related avoidance responses, empirically based challenges to early models of BPD have encouraged new treatment approaches. For example, recent evidence-based treatments no longer emphasize the need to "work through" client transference, projections, and split-off internal representations, as advocated by some psychoanalytic writers (e.g., Kernberg, 1975; Masterson, 1975; Stone, 2006). Instead, current treatments for BPD tend to involve interventions that focus on relational processing of early memories, emotional regulation training, cognitive-behavioral treatment of specific symptoms, and, in some cases, psychiatric medications (e.g., Choi-Kain, Finch, Masland, Jenkins, & Unruh, 2017; Lieb, Zanarini, Schmahl, Linehan, & Bohus, 2004). Importantly, borderline "acting-out" behaviors are more likely to be seen as coping strategies in the face of triggered distress than as ego-defensive or manipulative activities.

Whither BPD?

The relationship of this book to research and writing on BPD is complex. On the one hand, DRBs, and other avoidance responses such as dissociation and problematic substance use, are commonly among those with this diagnosis, and one of the most rigorous and empathic approaches to DRBs available to date—dialectical behavior therapy (DBT; Linehan, 1993, 2014)—is a treatment for BPD. On the other hand, many (probably most) of those who engage in DRBs do not meet diagnostic criteria for BPD, and not all people diagnosed with BPD are equally prone to DRBs (e.g., Bracken-Minor & McDevitt-Murphy, 2014; Brickman, Ammerman, Look, Berman, & McCloskey, 2014; Paris, 2007; Turner et al., 2015). The lack of a one-to-one concordance between BPD and DRBs can also be seen in their respective rates in the general population. For example, whereas self-injury, alone, has a prevalence rate of 6–20% (Briere & Gil, 1998; Klonsky, 2011) the rate of BPD is approximately 1–2% (ten Have et al., 2016).

Given this variability, DRBs should not be considered a specific symptom or pathognomonic indicator of BPD. Although the subjects of this book may self-injure, binge and purge, and engage in compulsive sexual behavior, they do not necessarily "have" the other symptoms and difficulties thought to be associated with BPD, whether idealization–devaluation, splitting, identity disturbance, black-and-white thinking, or boundary confusion (e.g., American Psychiatric Association, 2001). In fact, it is unlikely that DRB-involved individuals can be characterized by any single diagnosis, BPD or otherwise. To the extent that most people who engage in DRBs do not meet diagnostic criteria for BPD, borderline-focused interventions may not always be appropriate.

Impulse-Control Disorder(s)

The notion of impulse-control problems, reified in DSM-5 as *disruptive, impulse-control,* and *conduct disorder* diagnoses, is based on the idea that some people have insufficient abilities to control their urges and impulses, and thus behave in ways that nondisordered people would not. Such activities are generally categorized as risky to others or to oneself, and tend to violate social norms.

Behaviors often described in the psychiatric literature as involving inadequate impulse control, not all of which are listed as such in DSM-5, include aggressive outbursts, problematic or compulsive sexual behavior, compulsive hair pulling, repetitive fire setting, and impulsive stealing, as well as compulsive shopping and gambling. Because the "impulse-control" rubric is more descriptive than theoretically based, interventions are generally eclectic, focusing on treating the symptoms behaviorally (e.g., through emotional regulation skills development) or altering the neurochemistry of the response through psychiatric medication (Grant & Leppink, 2015).

There is nothing especially problematic about this model as a descriptive enterprise, except that it (1) can represent the medicalization of psychosocial problems, and (2) holds that DRBs arise due to inadequate neurological or psychological control, as opposed to the magnitude of the emotions that are to be controlled. For example, an individual who has a strong behavioral avoidance response to triggered memories of horrific trauma may not necessarily be suffering from impulse-control problems as much as responding to an internal state that most people would not be able to regulate. A reactive avoidance (RA) perspective, although also concerned with the development of emotional regulation capacities, equally highlights the role and strength of triggered memories and attachment schema. In such cases, it may be as important to help the client desensitize and process painful memories as it is to control what, for the client, has become uncontrollable.

Behavioral Addictions

As described by Grant, Potenza, Weinstein, and Gorelick (2010),

> the essential feature of behavioral addictions is the failure to resist an impulse, drive, or temptation to perform an act that is harmful to the person or to others. . . . The repetitive engagement in these behaviors ultimately interferes with functioning in other domains. In this respect, the behavioral addictions resemble substance use disorders. (p. 234)

Typical behaviors thought to be behavioral addictions include all of the activities described previously that can be seen as similar to substance use, except that they are referred to, for example, as "sex addiction," "food addiction," or "Internet addiction." The primary concern with this model is the assumption that all these behaviors necessarily share "common neurobiological processes" with one another, or, for that fact, substance addiction (Grant et al., 2010, p. 235).

Proponents of this model suggest that, like use of certain psychoactive substances, overinvolvement in euphoria-producing behaviors floods the pleasure circuitry of the brain (especially in the nucleus accumbens and orbito-frontal cortex) with dopamine and related neurotransmitters (Grant et al., 2010; Jentsch & Taylor, 1999; Volkow & Fowler, 2000). This process is highly reinforcing, leading to repetitive use of these behaviors to produce ongoing pleasure. Unfortunately, repeated activation of dopaminergic circuits leads to tolerance, as the brain responds to high levels of these neurotransmitters by down-regulating the associated receptor sites. As a result, the individual has to engage in more and more "addictive" activities to gain the same level of pleasure or well-being.

Although this research may partially explain why certain activities (e.g., problem gambling) are reinforced and can escalate over time, they are less informative about less overtly pleasurable behaviors, such as chronic self-injury, "impulsive" aggression, or repetitive suicide attempts. They also cannot explain why some individuals seem to become high-jacked by these brain dynamics, while others do not, or the absence of obvious withdrawal or tolerance effects among some so-called behavioral addictions, for example, compulsive sexual behavior or binge eating).

Perhaps most importantly, the addiction model has relatively little to say about the role of the most frequent correlates of so-called "addictive" behaviors: childhood abuse and neglect, attachment disturbance, high levels of emotional distress, and underdeveloped emotional regulation capacities.

Conduct and Oppositional Defiant Disorders

A final set of diagnosis commonly applied to those involved in DRBs are oppositional defiant and conduct disorders (ODD and CD, respectively), usually given to adolescents (as well as children) who routinely challenge authority and get "in trouble" on a regular basis. In the case of ODD, this can involve angry outbursts, frequent and intense arguments, interpersonal "vindictiveness," and "defiant" behavior in the face of authority (American Psychiatric Association, 2013). In CD, there may be more extreme rule breaking, physical aggression, fire setting, compulsive stealing, problematic sexual activity, and other "antisocial" behaviors (American Psychiatric Association, 2013). As predicted by the RA model, both ODD and CD have been linked to child maltreatment and attachment disturbance (American Psychiatric Association, 2013; Theule, Germain, Cheung, Hurl, & Markel, 2016), and ODD is commonly linked to emotional dysregulation (e.g., Cavanagh, Quinn, Duncan, Graham, & Balbuena, 2017).

Notably, because ODD/CD diagnoses are often applied in the face of "bad" behavior, they run the risk of pathologizing responses that are actually socially or adversity based. Further, many behaviors considered symptomatic of these disorders (e.g., angry outbursts, "impulsive" aggression, fighting, problematic sexual behavior, or stealing) may be more accurately seen as DRBs arising from easily triggered trauma memories or insecure attachment schema that are evoked in the context of impaired emotional regulation capacities. From an RA perspective, the treatment of ODD/CD may be most fruitful when it does not rely on external behavioral control or incarceration, but rather addresses the effects of child abuse and neglect and teaches emotional regulation and trigger management skills.

A Functional Analysis

Although all four of these diagnostic perspectives are helpful in understanding the inherent contradiction of repetitively engaged self- or other-endangering activities, most tend to overlook the distress reducing or compensatory aspects of such behaviors. In contrast, recent research—as well as the self-help literature, client disclosures during therapy, and lay postings on, for example, self-injury or compulsive gambling websites—indicate that most individuals who engage in these activities find them useful in reducing painful emotions, thoughts, and memories.

A focus on the specific reasons for problematic activities is important, because a greater understanding of exactly why people do such things can help the clinician to (1) target the true etiologies of problematic behavior; (2) avoid pathologizing, patronizing, or stigmatizing clients based on the seeming illogic of what they do under stress; and (3) provide explanations for otherwise impulsive or addictive behaviors that make intuitive sense to clients, thereby increasing their "buy-in" for specific treatment interventions.

Calling on several decades of research on the phenomenology and functions of behavioral avoidance (e.g., Briere, Hodges, & Godbout, 2010; Hayes, Luoma, Bond, Masuda, & Lillis, 2006; Linehan, 1993; van der Kolk, Perry, & Herman, 1991; Zeidner & Endler, 1996), this book introduces the RA model. This perspective does not consider self-injury or risky sexual behavior, for example, to necessarily be pathognomonic evidence of a medical or mental disorder, an addiction, or a borderline personality organization, but rather, as an adaptive—albeit often problematic—avoidance strategy. Importantly, RA interventions tend to focus on developing or increasing the client's strengths, capacities, and emotional survival skills, rather than her presumed deficits or psychological illness.

The RA Model

From an RA perspective, many of what are considered maladaptive, dys-functional, or self-defeating behaviors represent the individual's attempt to do what we would want him to do—to persevere despite sometimes great emotional pain, and to problem-solve rather than passively endure distress. These activities are reformulated in this book as DRBs, a more specific version of what was previously referred to as "tension reduction behaviors" (e.g., Briere, 1996; Briere & Scott, 2014). DRBs are viewed as immediately enacted avoidance responses to triggered distress and chal-lenged emotional regulation capacities that, although somewhat effective, have significant longer-term downsides.

The idea of functional avoidance is not the sole province of RA; related perspectives are found in, for example, acceptance and commit-ment therapy (ACT; Hayes, Strosahl, & Wilson, 2012) and DBT (Linehan, 1993). However, the RA model calls more directly on attachment and trauma theory, focuses extensively on trigger management, and devotes considerably more attention to emotional processing of both implicit and explicit memories.

Posttraumatic Stress and Dysphoria

The current trauma literature offers several principles that are relevant to the etiology and, ultimately, treatment of DRBs. The first is that expo-sure to upsetting events, especially those that overwhelm existing emo-tional regulation capacities, can create recurrent unwanted memories and enduring painful emotions. These posttraumatic states include intru-sive recollections and flashbacks, hyperarousal, overwhelming anxiety, depression, and anger (American Psychiatric Association, 2013) and, in some cases, powerful feelings of shame, guilt, emptiness, and self-hatred (Herman, 1992a,1992b). Although any highly adverse experience in life can likely produce these outcomes, they are most powerfully associated with complex trauma exposure, typically involving multiple forms of child abuse and neglect, often in the context of additional victimization experi-ences in adolescence or adulthood (Briere & Lanktree, 2012; Cloitre et al., 2009; Courtois & Ford, 2015; Herman, 1992a).

The second principle is that when faced with overwhelmingly nega-tive internal states, people almost always turn to some form of avoidance as a coping response. In general, there are two types of trauma-related avoidance. The first, *effortful avoidance,* involves attempts to avoid stimuli that otherwise might trigger distressing memories, thoughts, or feelings associated with adverse events (American Psychiatric Association, 2013). For example, a traumatized person might avoid certain people, places, sit-uations, or conversations that would activate painful memories of a past trauma. These responses are technically part of Criterion "C" of PTSD as described in DSM-5, but they are also found in many trauma survivors who do not meet criteria for a formal stress disorder.

The second, RA, involves the activities described in this book. They do not involve avoiding triggers, but, instead, are evoked in *response* to triggered posttraumatic distress and dysphoria. Some of these activities have been described as avoidance coping (Zeidner & Endler, 1996) or experiential avoidance (Hayes et al., 1996) in the literature, because they are invoked to decrease awareness of painful internal states, potentially allowing continued functioning in the face of significant emotional distress.

Functions of DRBs

Research and clinical experience (e.g., Briere & Gil, 1998; Dvir, Ford, Hill, & Frazier, 2014; Klonsky, 2007; Yates, 2004) suggests that DRBs typically pull attention or awareness away from emotional distress by providing one or more of the following:

- Distraction from painful internal states
- Self-soothing
- Distress-incompatible experiences
- Momentary interpersonal connection
- Displacement of negative internal experiences
- Communication of emotional distress in the face of desperation or social disconnection
- Relief from unwanted numbing or dissociation
- Self-punishment as a way to reduce guilt or shame
- An increased sense of control.

It might appear, then, that trauma and posttraumatic stress explain the existence of DRBs. Trauma can produce great distress, which then motivates activities that distract, soothe, or otherwise reduce awareness of emotional pain. There is empirical support for this possibility: As noted earlier, all of the DRBs described in this book are more prevalent among trauma survivors than others, and interventions that address traumatic stress are known to provide some assistance to individuals who engage in unsafe or problematic behaviors (e.g., Resick, Nishith, & Griffin, 2008).

However, there are significant problems associated with a trauma-only perspective on DRBs. First of all, not all people involved in self-injury, risky sexual activities, or binge eating, for example, report trauma histories (e.g., Linehan, 1993; Zanarini et al., 1997), and not all of those exposed to trauma exhibit significant negative effects (Bonanno, 2004), let alone engage in DRBs. In addition, treatment approaches that address trauma-related distress are not always especially helpful in the treatment of DRBs, either because trauma per se is not the only, or the most critical, issue (e.g., Linehan, 1993), or because, as described in Chapter 8, other factors interfere with trauma processing.

One hint that we may have to look beyond trauma alone comes from research indicating that not all prior adverse events correlate equally with adolescent or adult difficulties, including problem behaviors. Instead, most studies indicate that early trauma, especially child abuse, is more likely than later traumas to be associated with adult symptoms and problems (Briere & Rickards, 2007; Messman-Moore, Walsh, & DiLillo, 2010; Zlotnick et al., 2008). Furthermore, when studies include child neglect or caretaker disengagement as potential etiological factors, these phenomena tend to predict DRBs even more than do physical, psychological, or sexual abuse (Briere & Eadie, 2016; Briere, Runtz, Eadie, Bigras, & Godbout, 2017).

This raises a question: Why do early traumas matter more in the prediction of symptoms and problematic behaviors than later ones, and why is childhood emotional neglect at least as predictive of DRBs as child abuse, when neglect—although strongly associated with a range of psychological difficulties (Briere, Godbout, & Runtz, 2012; Hildyard & Wolfe, 2002)—is not generally defined as a trauma (American Psychiatric Association, 2013)?

Attachment-Related Difficulties

The answer may partially reside in what developmental psychologists and clinicians refer to as *parent–child attachment*. Attachment theory proposes that early caretaker responses to the child interact with the child's inborne biological systems to determine the extent to which proximity and connection (attachment) can occur. When the caretaker(s) is attached, attuned, nonviolent, and caring, the child can perceive safety, develop positive expectations of others, and learn important relational skills (Bowlby, 1988). Attachment theory further suggests that it is during the early attachment period that children first learns how to regulate their emotions and to develop a stable sense of self (Bowlby, 1973, 1977).

When caretaker responses to the child are characterized by abuse, rejection, loss, and/or emotional unavailability, however, insecure attachment is more likely (Baer & Martinez, 2006). In such instances, the child may not learn skills that otherwise would support the development and maintenance of secure relationships with others. Instead, he may generalize from early experiences of loss, lack of attunement, betrayal, or violence, and make incorrect, often blanket assumptions about the dangerousness of others in close relationships (Bowlby, 1988; Simpson & Rholes, 1998).

Attachment-related problems may be, in fact, the largest contributions—along with trauma—to the development of DRBs in adolescents and adults. Those who have negative attachment experiences are often subject to a host of painful memories, not only those involving classical trauma but also intrusive sensory and nonverbal recollections of early caretaker rejection, abandonment, or disengagement (e.g., Stern, 1985). As a result, it is not only traumatic stress that produces DRBs but also sensitivity to current relational stimuli (e.g., perceived rejection, betrayal, or nonresponsiveness) that trigger painful memories of early attachment disturbance. Thus, for example, the client with abandonment concerns or "authority issues" may perceive emotional unavailability or criticism in a current relationship, which then trigger powerful emotions and thoughts associated with early maltreatment or neglect, motivating seemingly out-of-proportion and problematic coping responses, including DRBs.

We may still not have enough information, however, to explain why some individuals engage in repetitive DRBs. As noted, there are many individuals who have experienced childhood trauma and/or attachment disturbance, who suffer as a result, yet do not engage in problematic avoidance responses, or who terminate such activities once their disadvantages become apparent. In order to complete this picture, there must be some phenomenon that mediates between triggered trauma/attachment memories and subsequent behavior—something that explains why one person might be triggered by current relational stimuli but not engage in DRBs, whereas another person would quickly turn to such behaviors.

Emotional Dysregulation

Research in the last decade or so suggests that this mediating variable is emotional regulation capacity (e.g., Briere et al., 2010; Dvir et al., 2014; Tull, Barrett, McMillan, & Roemer, 2007; Schore, 1994). Trauma or neglect early in life, especially when it produces attachment disturbance, is associated with later difficulties in tolerating and down-regulating painful emotional states (Levy, Johnson, Clouthier, Scala, & Temes, 2015). Although the reasons for this are not fully known, it is hypothesized that the unloved or maltreated child finds himself in an "emotional emergency": Continued abuse and/or neglect engenders high emotional distress, which must be addressed in order for the child to maintain homeostasis and ongoing functioning. But especially when these adversities occur early in life, the child may have insufficient psychological capacity to effectively reduce pain and dysphoria. In this overwhelming circumstance, the development of emotional regulation skills may be extremely difficult—in some sense akin to trying to learn how to swim while one is drowning.

Recent research also suggests that early trauma or neglect may reduce the brain's capacity to regulate stress, primarily by altering the functions of the hypothalamic–pituitary–adrenal (HPA) axis (Tarullo & Gunnar, 2006; Van Voorhees & Scarpa, 2004). When this dysregulated neurobiology is sustained, chronic emotional dysregulation typically results, leading to a nervous system that is more easily overwhelmed by distress (Schore, 2000).

Whether psychological or biological in nature, reduced emotional regulation capacity means that the formerly abused or neglected person is less able to tolerate—let alone regulate—painful internal experiences. This compromised capacity can easily lead to a reliance on avoidance strategies, whether "defensive exclusion" (Bowlby, 1988), in which the child reduces her awareness of psychological threats from caretaker(s), or later DRBs, in which the individual more generally learns to manage distress through seemingly "impulsive" or "maladaptive" behaviors (Schreiber, Grant, & Odlaug, 2012).

Activation–Regulation Balance

Summarizing the literature, it appears that triggered memory-related distress and insufficient emotional regulation are often both necessary in order for DRBs and other avoidance behaviors to occur at problematic levels. Importantly, neither distress nor inadequate emotional regulation capacity, alone, is usually sufficient to motivate clinically significant DRBs. For example, an individual might have a painful childhood history but have sufficient emotional regulation skills to keep from being overwhelmed by memories, and thus not need DRBs. Similarly, although less common, a person might have diminished emotional regulation capacities, but have a relatively benign childhood history, and therefore little potential for triggered distress, which would also result in an absence of DRBs.

Taken together, this research suggests that it is the balance between level of triggerable distress and existing emotional regulation capacities that determines whether an individual is internally overwhelmed and has to turn to DRBs. Throughout this book, this is referred to as the *activation–regulation balance,* a construct that will be called upon to explain not only avoidance behaviors but also the degree to which DRB-involved clients can tolerate exposure-based interventions.

The Integrated Model

In summary, the RA perspective suggests that a cascade of events lead to the development of DRBs and other problematic avoidance behaviors. This process may proceed as follows:

- The child is exposed to complex childhood traumas involving some combination of abusive, neglectful, and disengaged parenting.
- These negative experiences produce easily-triggered memories and associated emotional pain.
- In combination with genetic and neurobiological factors, this chronic and often unpredictable distress disrupts the natural parent–child attachment process, which generally requires environmental safety and stability.
- Subsequent insecure attachment and, potentially, dysregulated neurocircuitry precludes the development of emotional regulation capacities.
- When the (now older) person encounters stimuli in the current environment that are reminiscent of early adverse experiences—whether perceived rejection or lack of attunement, or more frank experiences of betrayal, abandonment, or maltreatment—she is triggered into childhood-era emotional distress.
- This emotional distress may be overwhelming or not, generally based on the client's activation–regulation balance.
- When the activation–regulation balance tilts toward overwhelming distress (i.e., when emotional pain exceeds available emotion regulation skills and neurobiology), the person is motivated to quickly (seemingly impulsively) invoke DRBs.

See Figure 1.1 for a graphical representation of this process.

Notably, all aspects of this model are supported in the attachment and/or trauma literature, whether it is the role of childhood trauma and neglect in DRBs (e.g., Homma, Wang, Saewyc, & Kishor, 2012), the additional importance of attachment disturbance in this process (e.g., Tatnell, Kelada, Hasking, & Martin, 2014), or the contributions of emotional dysregulation or intolerance in the etiology of maladaptive avoidance (e.g., Briere et al., 2010; van der Kolk, 1996).

Trigger Chaining

In some cases, triggering may be more complicated than described above. For example, a current adverse event (e.g., an assault) may lead to feelings (e.g., shame or anger) that then trigger recollections of a previous trauma (e.g., child sexual abuse) in which similar emotional reactions were present and encoded. When this occurs, RA theory refers to *trigger chains*: A cognitive or emotional response to a current event or stressor can serve as a stimulus that triggers similar emotional memories of one or more previous traumas. In the case of complex trauma, in which there are multiple traumas and, often, multiple painful attachment memories, there

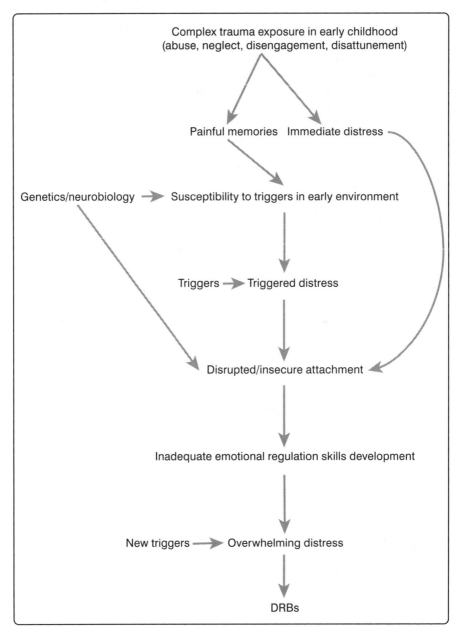

FIGURE 1.1. DRB development.

may be an extensive trigger chain: Thoughts/emotions associated with event 1 may trigger thoughts/emotions associated with event (or attachment experience) 2, which triggers thoughts/emotions associated with event or attachment experience 3, and so on. This is likely an explanation for why some individuals with a history of many traumas and attachment breaches have especially dramatic reactions to current stressors, ranging from more severe and complex outcomes (Briere, Kaltman, & Green, 2008; Cloitre et al., 2009) to greater risk of PTSD (Briere, Agee, & Dietrich, 2016; Karam et al., 2014). In fact, it appears that most traumatic stress disorders occur in the context of a history of multiple prior traumas; despite previous DSM criteria (American Psychiatric Association, 2000), it is surprisingly uncommon for them to arise from a single stressor alone (e.g., Briere, Agee, & Dietrich, 2016; Briere, Dias, Semple, Godbout, & Scott, 2017; Karam et al., 2014). In many cases, those with cumulative trauma and attachment disturbance suffer from insufficient emotional regulation capacities and experience a plethora of different triggered emotional responses to a range of previous adversities. As these emotions accumulate, interact, and trigger one another, the likelihood of a DRB increases.

Other Factors

Although triggered attachment or trauma memories are strongly implicated in the development of DRBs, there are additional phenomena that also can lead to problematic behaviors. These include not only the neurobiological aspects described earlier but also developmental disorders, such as autism, that motivate self-injury or related behaviors (Samson, Wells, Phillips, Hardan, & Gross, 2015), psychotic delusions or hallucinations that encourage harmful behaviors (Shawyer, Mackinnon, Farhall, & Copolov, 2008), and social systems or families that are highly stressful and demand perfection or aggression as problem-solving strategies (e.g., Butler, Lee, & Gross, 2007; Krahé, 2013). In some of these cases (e.g., autism), altered neurobiology may reduce emotional regulation capacities and lower the threshold for overwhelming distress (Mazefsky et al., 2013); in others, a mental disorder (e.g., schizophrenia or another psychotic disorder) may produce frightening internal states that overwhelm existing emotional regulation capacities (Lu, Mueser, Rosenberg, Yanos, & Mahmoud, 2017) or involve command auditory hallucinations to self-harm (Rogers, Watt, Gray, MacCulloch, & Gournay, 2002). For this reason, it is important that applications of the RA model include attention not only to attachment and trauma dynamics but also biological and social systems that impact the DRB-involved individual.

CHAPTER 2

An Overview of Specific Distress Reduction Behaviors

Based on the RA model described in Chapter 1, we review here a number of specific DRBs commonly seen among older adolescents and adults who were maltreated as children and/or were unable to form a secure attachment with their caretakers. Although the list is long, these responses tend to have several qualities in common:

- All have been implicated in the scientific or clinical literature as avoidance mechanisms, thought to operate by diverting attention away from painful emotions, "blocking" unwanted memories, providing distress-incompatible feelings, reducing unwanted dissociation, or otherwise altering awareness of painful internal states.
- Generally, these DRBs are triggered by phenomena in the person's current environment (e.g., perceived rejection or danger) that are reminiscent of early adverse events or processes; rarely do they occur in response to steady-state dysphoria alone.
- The presence of one or more DRBs often signals problems with emotional regulation. In such cases, even seemingly lower levels of triggered distress may overwhelm emotion regulation capacities, leading to DRBs that can appear "out of proportion," "excessive," or "overreactive." It is important to note that these social or clinical judgments are inaccurate: When distress exceeds capacity to regulate distress, it is, by definition, overwhelming—irrespective of how minor it may appear to others.

- Clinical experience suggests that DRBs are often, although not inevitably, cyclic:
  - The individual encounters an interpersonal stimulus in the current environment that is reminiscent of childhood trauma or attachment difficulties, which triggers intrusive and painful memories from the past.
  - When these states are intolerable, the person engages in a DRB as a way to reduce distress.
  - Unfortunately, DRBs are only temporarily effective and do not permanently eliminate the individual's painful emotions or negative thoughts, including shame, nor do they alter the presence of triggers in the environment. Furthermore, the DRB itself may produce additional dysphoria, shame, or guilt.
  - Avoidance responses such as DRBs can trigger *suppression effects* (see Chapter 6). Attempts to avoid thoughts, feelings, and memories, even when superficially successful, often lead to later, even more intense, intrusions of the suppressed thoughts, feelings, or memories (Briere, 2015).
  - Because nothing has actually changed as a result of the DRB, except that shame and guilt may have increased, and suppression effects may be in play, more DRBs may soon be necessary.
  - As a result, DRBs tend to reoccur and even accelerate over time. This cycle is presented graphically in Figure 2.1.

Major DRBs

Presented below are the most common forms of RA, although this list is not exhaustive. In fact, almost any behavior can be a DRB, to the extent that it is used to reduce awareness of triggered internal distress in the absence of sufficient emotional regulation capacity.

Self-Injurious Behavior

Dimitri began cutting on himself at age 13, first scratching his wrists with paper clips and broken glass after conflicts with his parents. He soon discovered that self-injury dramatically reduced his angry and anxious feelings, especially when he cut rather than scratched himself. By age 16, Dimitri was lacerating his inner arms and legs with razor blades several times a week, typically whenever he experienced guilt, shame, rejection, or criticism. He recently wrote in an essay for his freshman English class that "when the blade goes in, the pain goes out." Dimitri was psychologically and physically neglected by his

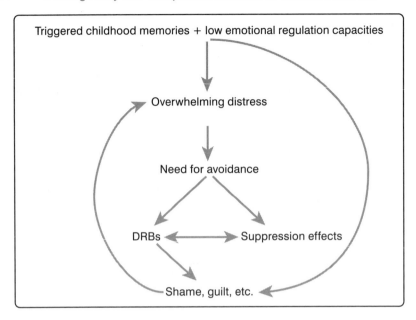

FIGURE 2.1. The DRB exacerbation cycle.

drug-addicted biological mother and sexually abused by his foster father. He states he has never attempted suicide, although he admits to suicidal ideation when he feels rejected or criticized.

Self-injurious behavior can be defined as intentional, self-inflicted bodily harm that is not primarily suicidal in nature, and that does not reflect normative social or cultural phenomena (e.g., Walsh, 2014; Walsh & Rosen, 1988). Although often referred to as *nonsuicidal self-injury* (NSSI; American Psychiatric Association, 2013), the more simple term *self-injurious behavior* is used here, in part because NSSI is increasingly considered a specific syndrome or disorder (Zetterqvist, 2015), whereas *self-injury* is a behavioral term that makes no assumptions about psychopathology. More importantly, some of those who self-injure are suicidal as well (e.g., Whitlock, Eckenrode, & Silverman, 2006; Grandclerc, De Labrouhe, Spodenkiewicz, Lachal, & Moro, 2016), and self-injury is a strong predictor of later suicide attempts (e.g., Asarnow et al., 2011; Linehan, 1993). At minimum, the fact that a client engages in self-injury is not a reliable indicator of the absence of concomitant suicidality; thus, the label NSSI may provide some degree of false assurance.

The research and clinical literature (e.g., Whitlock et al., 2006; Walsh, 2014) describes a range of self-injurious behaviors, including the following:

- Self-cutting
- Self-burning
- Self-stabbing or piercing
- Self-biting or chewing
- Picking at wounds or scabs
- Head banging
- Punching or hitting oneself or external objects (e.g., walls) with enough force to produce pain.

More rare types of self-injury include the following, although they tend to occur when other serious mental health issues (e.g., psychosis, mania) and/or extreme intoxication are also present (e.g., Favazza, 2001):

- Swallowing sharp objects that produce gastrointestinal pain or bleeding
- Eye enucleation
- Amputation
- Genital mutilation or castration
- "Autosurgery" (extensive and time-consuming cutting or "surgery," sometimes involving deliberate exposure of muscles, bones, or organs).

Although any area of the body can be the focus of self-injury, the most common areas are the inner arms or legs (Walsh, 2014). Some of those who self-injure do so on areas of the body that can be hidden with clothing, although others, especially those with strong interpersonal motives, may intentionally choose more visible sites. The age of onset for self-injury is typically early adolescence (e.g., Briere & Gil, 1998).

As predicted by the RA model, most of those involved in self-injury report that it reduces unwanted internal states, including anxiety, post-traumatic stress, self-loathing, emptiness, depression, and feelings of rejection or abandonment, and/or distracts from memories of childhood trauma or neglect (Briere & Gil, 1998; Brown, Comtois, & Linehan, 2002; Klonsky & Glenn, 2008). Notably, relief from dissociation also appears to be a common motive for self-injury (Briere & Eadie, 2016; Connors, 1996; Klonsky, 2007), especially when it addresses unwanted numbing, feelings of "deadness," or disconnection from reality. A number of studies suggest that self-injury, although effective in temporarily reducing awareness of some forms of distress, tends to be followed by feelings of shame and abnormality (e.g., Briere & Gil, 1998; Nixon, Cloutier, & Aggarwal, 2002), potentially leading to additional self-injury.

Self-injury is most common among trauma survivors (e.g., Ford & Gómez, 2015; Gratz, Conrad, & Roemer, 2002), especially those who were sexually abused as children (Dubo, Zanarini, Lewis, & Williams, 1997;

Glassman, Weierich, Hooley, Deliberto, & Nock, 2007), and those with inadequate emotional regulation capacities (Andover & Morris, 2014). Although some studies indicate that females are more likely to self-injure than males (e.g., Zlotnick, Mattia, & Zimmerman, 1999), others have found no gender differences at the multivariate level (e.g., Briere & Eadie, 2016).

Compulsive or Risky Sexual Behavior

> Michel, a 28-year-old man in long-term psychotherapy, describes himself as a "sex and drug addict." Sexually and emotionally abused as a child, he began initiating sex with other children in his early teens, followed by short-term relationships with older partners starting in later adolescence. By his own report, Michel has had at least 25 sexual partners within the last year, most of which were relatively anonymous. Many of these contacts occurred without protection and while under the influence of methamphetamine or alcohol. Michel states that "the sex usually isn't that good, to be honest," but that he seeks the physical contact and the momentary relief from loneliness and emptiness that sex sometimes provides.

DRBs subsumed under this category are generally defined according to their frequency, their indiscriminate nature, how many different partners are involved, and whether there are physical or social harms associated with the behaviors in question. Because some level of sexual behavior is obviously normative for all cultures, the cutoff for "too much" sex, the number of socially allowable sexual partners over a given period of time, and the amount of romance or commitment that must be involved, is relatively arbitrary. For the purposes of this book, application of the terms *compulsive* or *risky* sexual behavior is not based on whether consensual behaviors are socially acceptable, but rather on the extent to which they are invoked as an emotional avoidance strategy and have potential negative outcomes.

Compulsive sexual behavior is associated with childhood trauma in general but appears to be more common when childhood sexual abuse is part of the picture (Vaillancourt-Morel et al., 2015, 2016). As predicted by the RA model, it is also associated with attachment disturbance (e.g., Weinstein, Katz, Eberhardt, Cohen, & Lejoyeux, 2015) and difficulties with emotional regulation (e.g., Kafka, 2010).

Of all the DRBs, those involving sexuality are among the most associated with shame and guilt. This appears to be related to two phenomena: the frequent connection between sexual abuse and later compulsive sexual behavior, and the mixed feelings many cultures have regarding sexual behavior, particularly for specific groups. In the first case, problematic sexual behavior often occurs in the context of activated sexual abuse memories, which frequently carry with them powerful feelings of shame and badness. In fact, many clients who engage in sexually compulsive or risky behavior report being triggered into flashbacks or explicit recollections of sexual abuse before and during such sexual activities, resulting in a combination of current and childhood-era feelings and responses (Briere, 1996a). In addition, compulsive sexual behavior itself may be experienced as shameful, based on harsh social attitudes about who should be sexual, to what extent, and under what circumstances. For example, frequent sexual contacts with multiple partners may be viewed positively when it involves a heterosexual, white male (think James Bond), but may reinforce harmful stereotypes about "promiscuity" when engaged in by women or those with other sexual identities or orientations (Gentry, 1998; Spencer, 2016). As noted earlier, the additional, socially based shame associated with sexual DRBs may lead to even greater emotional distress and increase the risk of additional sexual DRBs.

There are several ways in which sexual behavior can be used to address triggered distress. Sex is typically pleasurable and thus to some extent distress-incompatible. For example, some people report that positive feelings associated with sexual contact or masturbation can be used to at least transiently neutralize negative feelings, thoughts, or memories (e.g., Smith, Kournos, & Meuret, 2014). Sexual contact also requires a degree of physical closeness, and some people report that briefly holding, or being held, soothes them in ways that address the effects of attachment deprivation (Briere, 1996). As well, sex may be used to counteract feelings of powerlessness, whether by increasing a sense of control over one's body or by seemingly controlling or impacting others (Monahan, Miller, & Rothspan, 1997; Walsh et al., 2013). Finally, pursuing, attracting, and sexually interacting with a partner may be an effective way to continuously distract oneself from negative internal states, as well as counter feelings of insecurity and unacceptability.

Because the goal of such behavior does not focus on a specific person per se, but rather on distress relief, compulsive sexual behaviors can be relatively indiscriminate in terms of the partners involved. Furthermore, the DRB-related—and thus temporary—nature of such activities may mean that high numbers of sexual contacts, or seemingly compulsive masturbation, are necessary to, as one client called it, "keep the dragons at bay." Finally, because insecure attachment often contributes to sexual DRBs (e.g., Weinstein et al., 2015), it may be preferable, in fact, *not* to have the same sex partner for long, since early experience may have taught the individual to avoid the dangers of intimacy or sustained relationships (Vaillancourt-Morel et al., 2016).

This pattern of indiscriminate contact with multiple partners over short periods of time for nonromantic reasons reinforces harsh cultural stereotypes regarding "sex addicts," "Don Juans," "party girls," and even more offensive descriptions of people assumed to be preoccupied with hedonistic pleasure. Unfortunately, in reality, those involved in sexual DRBs often experience the reverse of pleasure: Their avoidance strategy can be associated with desperation, social ostracism, and shame (e.g., Fong, 2006), risk of serious, even life-threatening diseases (Yoon, Houang, Hirshfield, & Downing 2016), and, based on the correlation between number of sexual partners and risk of sexual victimization (e.g., Krebs, Lindquist, Warner, Fisher, & Martin, 2007), an increased likelihood of sexual assault.

Notably, involvement in prostitution or other aspects of the sex industry (e.g., pornography, massage parlors, strip shows) typically is not a form of compulsive sexual behavior. Instead, these activities often reflect either victimization (e.g., sex trafficking, sexual acts forced or coerced by pimps or others) or a way to access money, drugs, food, or shelter in the relative absence of other options. In such cases, it is rare to see evidence of RA dynamics, whether building tension, compulsive behavior, or subsequent distress reduction. In fact, sexual behavior that is the result of exploitation or vastly narrowed economic or personal options is rarely perceived by those caught in the sex industry as sexual at all, let alone pleasurable (Farley, 2003).

Binge Eating

> Melissa, a 44-year-old architect and a member of Overeaters Anonymous, was sexually abused as a young child and later physically abused and neglected in foster care. The last day entered in her food log indicates that she ate one slice of dry toast at breakfast, a bag of three hamburgers and one order of fries while alone at lunch, a medium-size bag of potato chips while driving home, and a large pizza and an entire pie while watching TV in the evening. On the "triggers" section of her log, Melissa connects her binges to feeling anxious about work, feeling depressed about having binged on the hamburgers, and later, loneliness and self-loathing about being overweight and not having a romantic partner.

Binge eating refers to one or more episodes of seemingly compulsive overeating, often until uncomfortably full, even when not hungry, often in response to a triggered negative emotional state. The binge eater typically experiences a significant reduction in distress immediately upon eating, which then may be followed by shame or disgust.

From a clinical standpoint, there are two general categories of chronic binge eating: *binge-eating disorder* (BED), in which the person does not compensate for overeating, and *bulimia nervosa* (BN), in which compensatory purging (e.g., use of laxatives or vomiting) is an important feature (American Psychiatric Association, 2013). Although some people with BN are able to maintain a normal or lower weight, those involved in uncompensated bingeing (BED) are often overweight. Despite these differences, both BED and BN likely fall on the same spectrum of uncontrollable eating (Hay, Bacaltchuk, Stefano, & Kashyap, 2009).

Notably, not all those involved in purging are bulimic. There is also a "binge–purge" subtype of anorexia nervosa (Anorexia, Binge-Eating/Purging Type [ABPT]), in which anorectic food restriction coexists with instances of bingeing, purging, or both. Although DSM-5 discriminates BED, BN, and ABPT, all three of these diagnoses overlap to some extent in terms of symptomatology, and some clients cycle through these different eating patterns over time. As a result, we will generally refer to bingeing–purging in this book rather than bulimia or anorexia per se.

The focus on bingeing and purging is also important, because it should be discriminated from *anorexia nervosa, restricting type* (American Psychiatric Association, 2013). This eating pattern is not considered to include DRBs, nor is it especially linked to childhood trauma or attachment disturbance (see a review by Briere & Scott, 2007). Not only does its etiology appear to differ from that of bulimic or anorectic bingeing and purging, food restriction is usually not a triggered avoidance response; it is instead an ongoing process involving intentional weight loss, fear of gaining weight, preoccupation with thinness, and, in most cases, a distorted body image (Morris & Twaddle, 2007). Because triggering and reduced emotional regulation are not central aspects of the (purely) restricting form of anorexia nervosa, the interventions described in this book may be of limited usefulness for this form of disordered eating.

Although genetics may play a significant role (Trace, Baker, Peñas-Lledó, & Bulik 2013), the modern literature on binge eating strongly supports an RA perspective. A number of studies indicate that those who eat excessively, as well as those who purge afterward, are more likely to have been abused or neglected as children (see the review by Briere & Scott, 2007), to have more attachment difficulties (e.g., Zachrisson & Skårderud, 2010) and problems with emotional regulation (e.g., Gianini, White, & Masheb, 2013), to occur after significant dysphoria, including depression, emptiness, low self-esteem, and posttraumatic stress (e.g., Polivy & Herman, 1993; Stice, 2002), and to be followed by disgust or shame (Lynch, Everingham, Dubitzky, Hartman, & Kasser, 2000). As expected, many report that their overeating responses are triggered by negative relational stimuli that activate unwanted emotional states (e.g., Ansell, Grilo, & White, 2012).

Reactive Aggression

Nanda, a 28-year-old man, is currently incarcerated in a county jail on two counts of simple assault. He says he has always had "anger issues," and that he "flies off the handle" at "any damn thing." He has been arrested several times in the past, usually in the context of a verbal altercation with another man that becomes violent. When not triggered into rage, however, Nanda is a seemingly pleasant and likable person who has multiple friends. During his trial, his lawyer suggested several potentially mitigating factors for his latest offense, including his teenage abandonment by a physically and emotionally abusive alcoholic father, who on at least one occasion beat Nanda so badly that he was hospitalized overnight.

Reactive aggression is defined here as aggressive outbursts or seemingly impulsive violence against others that is not planned or proactively intended, and that is usually triggered by a negative relational event. In many cases, the reactively aggressive person experiences guilt, shame, or fears of abandonment after the incident, only to respond violently again in the near future. Notably, this definition does not include planned or premeditated forms of aggression or violence (Dodge, 1991).

Often linked to BPD, intermittent explosive disorder, or conduct disorder (American Psychiatric Association, 2013), reactive aggression frequently shares the same cascade of events with other DRBs, such as self-injury or binge eating. Specifically, it is often associated with a sudden upsurge of feelings (e.g., anger), typically triggered by experiences of perceived rejection, betrayal, dismissal, unfairness, or criticism (Blair & Lee, 2013; Smart Richman & Leary, 2009), leading to verbal, physical, or sexual aggression, outbursts, bullying, and other behaviors that are disproportionate to their superficial causes (e.g., Ardino, 2012; Ford, Chapman, Connor, & Cruise, 2012; Kerig, 2013; Silvern, 2011).

Importantly, many people have good reasons for anger, including those exposed to systemic social discrimination, victimization, and marginalization. Similarly, the injustice and unfairness of exploitation, childhood abuse, and adult interpersonal violence almost inevitably lead to angry feelings, whether or not their expression is allowed or supported. Thus, being appropriately angry, even if anger is a predominant emotion, is not a sign of an impulse control or personality disorder. At the same time, however, some people can be triggered and dysregulated by sudden posttraumatic intrusions of anger, and may be transiently dangerous to others as a result. Thus, the question of whether anger is a valid treatment target will depend on whether it is an unwanted triggered phenomenon that endangers the client and, potentially, others, or a contextually appropriate reaction that may in fact even fuel prosocial behaviors, such as self-assertion and social action.

Although anger is an obvious aspect of reactive aggression, clinical experience suggests that other thoughts or feelings (e.g., fear of abandonment, posttraumatic stress, feelings of inadequacy) also may be present. In fact, violence may sometime arise from triggered emotions associated with early insecure attachment or trauma exposure (e.g., Dutton, 1998; Godbout et al., 2017), frequently in the context of insufficient affect regulation (Babcock, Jacobson, Gottman, & Yerington, 2000).

Notably, there are often multiple reasons for aggression, including broad social factors that allow or encourage violence against those with lesser social status or power (e.g., Krahé, 2013; White, Koss, & Kazdin, 2011), the clinician should be careful to parcel out the multiple motives underlying, for example, child abuse, partner violence, or sex or hate crimes. He or she should also be cautious about relying entirely on an RA perspective in forensic or clinical settings when other variables may be more relevant.

Triggered Suicidal Behavior

> Tamara, a 24-year-old woman, was recently admitted to an ER for overdosing on aspirin and muscle relaxants. This is her third ER admission, each of which occurred immediately after a conflict with a romantic partner. As in previous instances, Tamara was extremely upset and *verbalizing* suicidal intent upon admission, but appeared calm several hours later, stating that she and her boyfriend had "made up" over the phone and that she wanted to go home. Raised by a seemingly caring but overwhelmed and emotionally disengaged single mother, Tamara was episodically sexual abused by her brother and an uncle between ages 9 and 12.

Triggered suicidal behavior can be defined as suicide threats and attempts that occur when an experience of conflict, betrayal, abandonment, or rejection triggers painful memories or negative attachment schemas, somewhat equivalent to what are described as *parasuicidal* attempts in DBT (Linehan, 1993). Clinicians often characterize these suicidal behaviors as impulsive, dramatic, or "gestures," that are assumed to be employed for secondary gain (see a review by Heilbron, Compton, Daniel, & Goldston, 2010). Although modern researchers and clinicians appropriately disparage this perspective as dismissive and inaccurate (Heilbron et al., 2010) and note that such behavior can, in fact, be injurious, if not lethal, psychiatry and clinical psychology have a long tradition of devaluing triggered suicidality and framing it in the context of personality disorder and manipulative behavior.

In contrast, this suicidal response may be best understood as a form of DRB, in which the "impulsive" nature of such behavior reflects rapidly engaged avoidance responses to triggered, potentially overwhelming emotional states (e.g., Zouk, Tousignant, Seguin, Lesage, & Turecki, 2006). Similarly, the "dramatic" and "manipulative" aspects of triggered suicidality may at least partially reflect interpersonal helplessness and proximity-seeking in the face of activated feelings of abandonment, rejection, disengagement, or loss (Linehan, 1993). One might reflect, for example, on the amount of desperation and dysphoria necessary for an individual to engage in potentially life-threatening behavior "just" to receive attention or nurturance from others.

It is important to note that suicidality that is not triggered also can arise from trauma. For example, survivors of rape, torture, and other forms of adult trauma also are at increased risk of suicide attempts (e.g., Ferrada-Noli, Asberg, Ormstad, Lundin, & Sundbom, 1998; Kilpatrick, Edmunds, & Seymour, 1992; O'Neill et al., 2014), in many cases because trauma-related depression and posttraumatic hyperarousal, shame, and other outcomes are sufficiently aversive that suicide may appear to be the only solution (e.g., Briere, Godbout, & Dias, 2015; Bryan, Rudd, & Wertenberger, 2014). Such responses are reactive as well, but they typically do not involve triggered emotional memories or feelings associated with childhood abuse, neglect, or attachment issues. Instead, the precipitating emotional state originates in older adolescence or adulthood, and the goal of suicide is often permanent escape from pain.

To make things even more complicated, however, clinicians are sometimes confronted with those whose childhood traumas or attachment difficulties are triggered and compounded by exposure to later traumas, a form of which was described earlier as *trigger chaining*. Although this is a more complicated scenario, such complex trauma survivors are, by definition, experiencing triggered suicidality. However, the trigger in this case is a current adversity that is reminiscent of an earlier one (e.g., rape triggering memories of childhood sexual abuse, or a current relationship breakup triggering early experiences of abandonment), such that both contribute to suicide risk.

Ultimately, triggered suicidality is one of the most complex of the DRBs, because there are many motives for suicidal behavior (Nock et al., 2008); some involve triggered attachment- and trauma-related emotions and schema, and others do not. For this reason, further assessment is important to determine whether a given act represents a DRB or, instead, more classic suicidality. For example, one might ask: Is this attempt or threat based on

- depression, PTSD, or a desire to escape from chronic and severe psychological or physical pain,
- a current interpersonal event triggering early memories and distress, or
- a combination of both?

A functional analysis of triggered suicidality suggests treatment approaches that differ to some extent from what are typically employed to prevent less trauma- or attachment-related attempts. Although the latter generally requires intervening in depression, cognitive distortions, inadequate coping, or PTSD, treatment of triggered suicidal behavior may also include trigger management (see Chapter 7); processing of painful attachment-level memories and cognitions involving rejection, nonsupport, and loss; and facilitating the development of emotional regulation skills.

Other DRBs

In addition to the major forms of distress reduction described earlier, there are a number of other activities or behaviors that reflect the same underlying processes and that are often characterized as addictions, compulsive behavior, or impulsivity. These include excessive involvement in gambling, shopping, stealing, and Internet use, as well as fire setting, compulsive hair pulling, and skin picking.

Problem Gambling

Roberto, a 32-year-old physician, first began playing poker with friends in medical school. Severely emotionally neglected as a child, and generally prone to anxiety and insecurity, he soon discovered that gambling made him feel confident and, when winning, euphoric. By the time he graduated, Roberto was gambling on an almost a daily basis, for higher and higher stakes, but was losing more than winning. By the end of his residency, he was financially insolvent and had lost most of his friends due to unpaid debts. Following a suicide attempt, he began attending Gamblers Anonymous and seeing a therapist. Roberto now abstains from gambling but continues to fantasize about winning a fortune and redeeming himself to others.

Often referred to as "compulsive," "pathological," or "addictive" gambling, this DRB occurs when a person bets or gambles on a frequent and often escalating basis, and is not able to stop doing so despite serious personal and social consequences, including bankruptcy, major losses, and disrupted relationships. Problem gambling closely parallels the antecedents and phenomenology of other DRBs: (1) It is often associated with abuse, neglect, and other adverse childhood experiences (Scherrer et al., 2008; Sharma & Sacco, 2015), as well as insecure attachment (Di Trani, Renzi, Vari, Zavattini, & Solano, 2017; Testa et al., 2017) and emotional regulation problems (Di Trani et al., 2017; Williams, Grisham, Erskine, & Cassedy, 2012); (2) it is invoked to address "unpleasant feelings such as stress, depression, loneliness, fear, or anxiety" (California Council on Problem Gambling; *www.calpg.org/cravings-and-triggers*); (3) it results in excitement and distress relief (Wood & Griffiths, 2007; Wood, Gupta, Derevensky, & Griffiths, 2004), yet (4) it is often followed by feelings of shame or regret (Wood & Griffiths, 2007; Yi & Kanetkar, 2011).

Among other characteristics, DSM-5 notes that the compulsive gambler also

- Needs to gamble for higher and higher stakes in order to maintain positive feelings.
- Experiences restlessness and/or irritability when attempting to stop.
- Is typically unable to reduce or quit gambling.
- Is preoccupied with thoughts and memories of gambling.
- Suffers relational, social, occupational, or educational losses due to gambling.

Compulsive Theft

Dyani is a 36-year-old actor, recently arrested for a third time for stealing cosmetics from a department store. Extremely embarrassed, she denies the theft despite store camera evidence. She eventually admits to her therapist that this shoplifting episode was related to the breakup of a 2-year relationship, and an unsuccessful attempt to reconcile with her father, who was physically aggressive and emotionally unavailable when she was young.

Also known as *kleptomania,* compulsive theft or shoplifting is described in DSM-5 as an impulse control disorder that involves (1) a general inability to resist the impulse to steal things that are not personally needed or valuable, (2) a building sense of pressure to steal that is most intense just before the theft occurs, and (3) a sense of pleasure or relief immediately following the theft (American Psychiatric Association, 2013, p. 478). In most cases, stealing is not planned ahead of time and occurs "on impulse," often in the context of stress or a trigger. The objects stolen are rarely wanted or desired by the person, could typically be paid for, and are often either thrown away afterward or hoarded with other stolen objects. Relative to other DRBs, compulsive stealing, like reactive aggression, is more likely to involve contact with the criminal justice system, which is generally more concerned with administering penalties than providing mental health assistance.

Notably, as per DSM-5 criteria, compulsive shoplifting or stealing does not include behaviors arising from poverty or other social conditions that might motivate stealing of food or other needed supplies. Instead, the thrill of taking something without detection appears to produce distress-incompatible and distracting states. Supporting the notion that compulsive stealing is unrelated to the worth of the items stolen, a number of wealthy people have been caught shoplifting objects of minor value, such as cosmetics, pieces of clothing, and inexpensive jewelry (e.g., Marikar, 2008).

Problematic Internet Use

> Donald, a 17-year-old youth, is currently in therapy at a specialized treatment center for "Internet addiction." By his own report, he usually spends at least 10–12 hours of screen-time a day in his bedroom, in addition to his part-time attendance at a college for computer program coders. Chronically abused as a child, and not comfortable in real-time social interactions, Donald devotes most of his waking hours to massively multiplayer online role playing games, first-person shooter games, conspiracy websites, and, increasingly, Internet pornography. He becomes irritable and upset if kept from his computer, to the point that his adoptive parents have stopped insisting he do other things. Donald denies that this is a problem, noting that his multiplayer peers and fellow students are all online as much or more than he is.

Internet addiction can be defined as excessive and preoccupying Internet-related behavior that facilitates distress avoidance but interferes with daily life (e.g., Byun et al., 2009). The specific diagnosis of Internet addiction was unsuccessfully suggested for inclusion in DSM-5, but will be included in 11th edition of the *International Classification of Diseases* (ICD-11, beta draft; World Health Organization, 2016), based on literature documenting excessive use, distress upon terminating Internet activities, tolerance (i.e., requiring increasing amounts of Internet use to gain the same distress-reducing effect), and continued use despite negative repercussions such as poor achievement and social isolation (Block, 2008). The DSM proposal suggested three subtypes: excessive gaming, sexual preoccupations, and e-mail/text messaging. Of these, compulsive Internet pornography use (Love, Laier, Brand, Hatch, & Hajela, 2015) appears to be the most common (Meerkerk, van den Eijnden, & Garretsen, 2006), and may represent a form of compulsive sexual behavior (masturbation) for which the Internet is primarily a delivery device. In any case, studies of compulsive pornography use highlight its use as a distraction from dysphoria and as a way to generate distress-incompatible states (e.g., arousal, orgasm), which are often followed by guilt and shame (Laier & Brand, 2017; Love et al., 2015; Twohig & Crosby, 2010).

Like other DRBs, compulsive Internet use often occurs in the context of insecure attachment (e.g., Eichenberg, Schott, Decker, & Sindelar, 2017), emotional regulation disturbance (Yildiz, 2017), and the need to avoid chronic negative emotional states (García-Oliva & Piqueras, 2016).

Compulsive Buying/Shopping

Lilly, a 48-year-old woman, is struggling to keep a house that she has owned for 8 years. Although employed as an airplane mechanic for over a decade, she has been unable to keep up on mortgage payments and property taxes, and is being pursued by her bank and state taxation board for late and insufficient payments. When a federal Marshal came to her house to serve a foreclosure notice, he discovered a home filled with unopened or seemingly unused merchandise, including piles of books, clothing, canned food, and boxes of shoes. Lilly states that she shops online whenever she feels upset or sad, and that she can't stop doing so. During the shopping and purchasing process, she briefly feels calm and slightly euphoric, but she is plagued by shame and guilt afterwards.

Compulsive buying is described as "chronic, repetitive purchasing behavior that occurs as a response to negative events or feelings" (O'Guinn & Faber, 1989, p. 149), typically involving excessive acquisition of unneeded products, even when they cannot be afforded (Hoyer & MacInnis, 2007). For all but the most affluent, compulsive buying can result in unsustainable debt and sometimes bankruptcy (Kellett & Bolton, 2009). As is true of other DRBs, compulsive shopping often begins with a buildup of tension and distress after a triggering interpersonal event, followed by relief during the purchase process (Black, 2007), and later postpurchase guilt (Workman & Paper, 2010). For some people, there appear to be four distinct phases of compulsive buying, each of which is distracting and rewarding: (1) anticipation, (2) preparation, (3) shopping, and (4) spending (Black, 2007).

As predicted by the RA model, those involved in compulsive buying are more likely to have a history of childhood trauma (Sansone, Chang, Jewell, & Rock, 2013), as well as difficulties with emotional regulation (Claes et al., 2010; Williams & Grisham, 2012).

Fire Setting

Vito is currently incarcerated for setting a fire that destroyed 38 acres of forest in a national park. He was well known to fire marshals and investigators, with a previous conviction for fire setting as an adolescent and several suspected fires since then. He had been photographed by arson investigators at the scene of two abandoned house fires, although they were unable to link him to either blaze.

Abused and neglected as a child, Vito first set a fire at age 10 and discovered that the experience transiently replaced his anxiety and anger with excitement and sexual arousal. Socially avoidant, he often fantasizes in great detail about setting fires, and, in some cases, fighting them, especially after stressful or upsetting interpersonal interactions.

Compulsive fire setting, or *pyromania,* is "characterized by recurrent failure to resist impulses to set fires, tension before setting the fire and satisfaction and relief after doing it" (Blanco et al., 2010, p. 1219). This behavior pattern is separate from *arson,* which involves setting fires for financial gain, vengeance, or some other external motive. As with other DSM-5 impulse-control disorders, compulsive fire setting is characterized by growing tension or emotional arousal before the act, and relief or pleasure during the process. Typically, the affected individual is fascinated with fire and fire setting, including the paraphernalia involved. As noted in DSM-5, compulsive firesetters are often regular "watchers" of local fires, may trigger fire alarms in order to observe arriving fire trucks and personnel, and generally are preoccupied with firefighting institutions and equipment—to the extent that a small minority even become firefighters (pp. 476–477).

As predicted by the RA model, compulsive fire setting is more common among those who were abused or neglected as children (Gannon & Pina, 2010), and those with emotional dysregulation and attachment problems (Gannon, Ó Ciardha, Doley, & Alleyne, 2012).

Hair Pulling ("Trichotillomania") and Skin Picking ("Excoriation")

Ailene, a 34-year-old assistant professor of textile science at a state university, has engaged in compulsive hair pulling for over a decade. She wears a wig to cover multiple bald patches and areas of short, newly grown hair. Ailene feels unable to control her behavior, which usually involves pulling one to several hairs out of her scalp in a very specific, almost ritualistic way, after which she chews the hair and then throws it away. This behavior typically starts when she is triggered into memories of a painful childhood, which then activate feelings of anxiety, insecurity, and inwardly directed anger. She experiences a strong sense of relief during and briefly after hair pulling but is then consumed by shame.

Variously categorized as impulse-control disorders or part of an obsessive–compulsive disorder, these DRBs involve compulsively picking at the skin or scabs (excoriation) or pulling hair from the scalp or body (trichotillomania), sometimes both together (Stein et al., 2010). In some cases, excoriation is classified as a form of self-injury, especially when picking has produced significant wounds that are prevented from healing. When compulsive hair pulling is severe, the individual may present with obvious bald patches on the scalp, eyebrows, and/or beard. As per other DRBs, there is usually increasing tension or anxiety before the activity and relief afterward (Chamberlain, Menzies, Sahakian, & Fineberg, 2007; Stein et al., 2010). Although there may be a genetic influence (e.g., Zuchner et al., 2006), both trichotillomania and excoriation are more common among those abused as children (Özten et al., 2015), and both have been linked to emotional regulation problems (e.g., Arabatzoudis, Rehm, Nedeljkovic, & Moulding, 2017; Roberts, O'Connor, & Bélanger, 2013).

Episodic, Nonspecific DRBs

Quang is a 26-year-old man who lives in his parents' home and works part-time at a vape shop. A self-identified "partier," he occasionally uses ecstasy, smokes cannabis daily, and has frequent, brief, and often tumultuous relationships with women. He is liked by his friends, although they note that he often "takes things too far," for example, driving too fast, often recklessly, yelling and throwing things during arguments, abruptly crossing streets in the middle of fast-moving traffic, and taking unnecessary chances when snowboarding or rock climbing. When asked about his risky behavior by a friend, he states that he just needs to "take it to the edge" when he is frustrated, angry, or bored. Quang was adopted at age 5, and little is known about his earlier life, other than he was removed from his substance-addicted biological parents for severe physical and psychological neglect, and an unspecified "unhealthy family environment."

Episodic, nonspecific DRB use typically involves a wide range of simultaneously engaged distress avoidance behaviors, many of which involve thrill seeking and dramatic behavior, as well as DRBs that especially distract from triggered distress. These include not only reckless driving and involvement in other dangerous or risky activities but also lower-level or episodic involvement in avoidance activities described previously, including less discriminant sexual behavior, seemingly "impulsive" aggression, and substance use. In many cases, individuals involved in nonspecific DRBs, by definition, do not utilize one or two types of avoidance, nor are they typically unable to discontinue any given DRB when necessary. Instead, they invoke any of a number of avoidance behaviors when distressed or, in some cases, bored. Although this generalized DRB style is typically associated with RA antecedents and dynamics, research also suggests the influence of genetics and neurobiology (often involving dopamine and serotonin), especially when there is a preponderance of thrill- or sensation-seeking behaviors (Netter, Hennig, & Roed, 1996; Norbury, Manohar, Rogers, & Husain, 2013).

Non-DRBs That Involve Maladaptive Coping

A characteristic aspect of DRBs is that distress relief arises directly from the behavior performed, generally because the action itself distracts or redirects attention, soothes, or provides distress-incompatible states. There are two major avoidance strategies, however, that do not operate in this fashion: substance use and dissociation. Although, in the case of the former, the euphoria associated with drug or alcohol consumption can negate adverse emotions, the primary function of each of these responses is to reduce awareness, either by numbing feelings or by altering access to integrated experience. Notably, in the case of substance use, the behaviors involved (pursuing drugs or alcohol; drinking, ingesting, or injecting) generally do not directly produce the effect, as is the case for DRBs. Instead, these behaviors are the delivery mechanism for the effects: Drinking, for example, administers alcohol to the gut, then to the nervous system, and the alcohol, typically not the behavior, alters internal experience.

In this regard, substance use exerts its avoidance effects through the induction of anesthesia or euphoria that, by virtue of its specific chemistry, overrides or numbs unwanted feelings. Occasionally, in fact, related neurochemical responses may begin even prior to the consumption of the substance, for example, when preparing a drug (e.g., heroin) before injection, breaking the seal on a bottle of whisky, or merely looking at a glass of wine produces momentary calm or well-being. In such cases, substance preparation or sensory exposure is thought to trigger a conditioned emotional response, generated by the association between these actions and subsequent euphoria or distress reduction.

Similarly, dissociation is often associated with distress reduction (Dalenberg et al., 2012), but it is rarely a directly chosen behavior, and it does not provide many of the functions associated with DRBs. For example, dissociation generally does not distract or soothe; instead, it directly alters awareness either by numbing feelings or by compartmentalizing experience.

Although these two avoidance response are not defined as DRBs, they are included in this book because they, too, are often used to reduce negative emotional states and experiences, and thus may be invoked simultaneously with DRBs. As well, in both cases, they may complicate, or even motivate, distress reduction activities.

Dissociation

Ashley is a 25-year-old woman with an extensive history of childhood maltreatment, including early neglect, followed by sexual abuse at the hands of a foster parent. She lived on the streets for several years in her early adolescence, generally by trading sex for food, shelter, and drugs, but was able to (in her words) "clean up" in her early 20s and complete a course in dental assisting. She has been fired from two dental offices, in both cases because of absent-mindedness, inattention, losing things, and times when she has been found staring into space, largely unresponsive to staff or patients around her. Ashley's therapist has diagnosed her with depersonalization–derealization disorder, but also notes what appear to be brief fugue states and related amnestic periods.

Dissociation can be defined as a defensive reduction or alteration in awareness of one's thoughts, feelings, perceptions, and/or memories (e.g., American Psychiatric Association, 2013), often in response to a traumatic event (Dalenberg et al., 2012) or insecure attachment (Lyons-Ruth, Dutra, Schuder, & Bianchi, 2006). Although there are a number of dissociative responses, including dissociative identity disorder and dissociative amnesia, the most common are *disengagement* (e.g., "spacing out"), *emotional constriction* (e.g., reduced or numbed emotional response), and *depersonalization–derealization* (experiences of unreality and/or separation or detachment from one's body) (American Psychiatric Association, 2013; Briere, Weathers, & Runtz, 2005; Dell & O'Neil, 2009).

In general, dissociation functions as a way to reduce awareness of emotional (and sometimes physical) pain to tolerable levels, at which point it no longer overwhelms. As such, it is a commonly used coping technique, albeit one that is problematic to the extent that it decreases awareness or attention when it is most needed (i.e., during danger), blocks emotional processing of memories, and produces symptoms or states that interfere with daily living. As well, because of the suppression effect described in Chapter 6, dissociated emotions and memories may recur as intrusive symptoms at later moments in time (e.g., Elliott & Briere, 1995), potentially motivating even more avoidance.

As expected, there is a substantial literature linking dissociation to a range of traumas, especially child abuse (e.g., Briere et al., 2005; Sar, Akyüz, & Doğan, 2007), but also sexual and physical assaults (e.g., Elliott, Mok, & Briere, 2004; Schalinski, Elbert, & Schauer, 2011), and combat exposure (e.g., Bremner et al., 1992; Maguen et al., 2009). Notably, although a common risk factor, a history of adverse events alone is often insufficient to produce significant lasting dissociation (Briere, 2006). As is true for DRBs, the likelihood of dissociation increases when there is also early attachment disturbance, perhaps especially of the "disorganized" type (Briere, Runtz, Eadie, Bigras, & Godbout, 2018; Main & Morgan, 1996; Bureau, Martin, & Lyons-Ruth, 2010) and inadequate emotional regulation or tolerance (e.g., Briere, 2006).

Paradoxical Effects of Dissociation

Notably, the effects of dissociation can vary according to type and intensity. At low to moderate levels, disengagement and emotional constriction appear to be relatively effective in temporarily decreasing awareness of, or separation from, unwanted internal states. Yet other forms of dissociation, for example, derealization and depersonalization, may not only serve some distress-reducing functions, for some, but may also be experienced as aversive, even at lesser levels. For example, Spiegel (2017) notes that symptoms of depersonalization–derealization disorder "are almost always distressing and, when severe, profoundly intolerable. Anxiety and depression are common. Some patients fear that they have irreversible brain damage or that they are going crazy. Others obsess about whether they really exist or repeatedly check to determine whether their perceptions are real."

Probably for this reason, some individuals report using DRBs, especially self-injury, to decrease dissociation (e.g., Klonsky, 2007). For example, some who self-harm appear to use the associated pain to reorient or "wake up" from the unwanted effects of numbing, depersonalization, or derealization (Briere & Eadie, 2016). The effectiveness of self-injury-related pain as a way of altering dissociation is described not only in research but also on some self-injury support websites (e.g., *www.lifesigns.org.uk*), and in popular songs—for example, "I hurt myself today, to see if I still feel. I focus on the pain, the only thing that's real" ("Hurt"; Reznor, 1994).

These paradoxical effects may reflect, in part, what Hebb (1955) referred to as the "optimal arousal curve": Too little or too much emotional arousal is experienced as unpleasant, leading to anxiety, whereas optimal (intermediate) arousal is perceived as neutral or pleasurable. In the case of dissociation, high dissociation can lead to low arousal and is therefore distressing, whereas intermediate levels may reduce trauma- or attachment-level distress without producing hypoarousal-related anxiety.

In this regard, it is possible that high emotional distress can motivate dissociation as a defensive response, but if the dissociation is too great or has unwanted side effects (e.g., the dislocation or "deadness" of depersonalization), the individual ultimately may need to invoke a DRB to down-regulate dissociation. In this sense, dissociation and dissociation–disruption may be used simultaneously, titrating the former to an intermediate state in which it is effective against distress but is not distressing itself (Briere & Eadie, 2016).

Problematic Substance Use

> Priya, a 31-year-old woman, is currently in residential treatment for polysubstance use, primarily methamphetamine, cocaine, and alcohol abuse, but also occasionally Oxycontin, "spice," and marijuana. She first used drugs in early adolescence, which she relates to extensive sexual abuse by her stepfather and his friends at that time. Although highly intelligent, her substance use has kept her from pursuing a higher-level education or holding jobs for more than a few months at a time. Staff and others are strongly invested in Priya's well-being, frequently describing her as "sweet" and "smart." They also note, however, that she has a low tolerance for stress or conflict, and seems to use drugs to regulate her easily triggered distress. As one counselor put it, "She's fine when everything's fine."

The term *substance abuse* is not used in DSM-5, which instead refers to mild, moderate, or severe levels of "substance use disorder"—defined by the extent to which the recurrent use of alcohol or other psychoactive substances is associated with impaired control, social problems, risky use, and physiological issues of tolerance and withdrawal (American Psychiatric Association, 2013). Because the term *disorder* locates substance use in the medical domain, despite its many psychological and functional aspects, in this book *problematic substance use* is employed to indicate the repeated use of psychoactive substances (including alcohol) that produces significant negative outcomes, whether social, psychological, or physical.

Like DRBs and dissociative responses, substance use is a commonly employed avoidance response, one that serves to numb painful internal states or distract from distress by producing distress-incompatible euphoria. Those exposed to traumatic events—especially childhood maltreatment—are considerably more likely to use psychoactive substances (Ouimette & Brown, 2003; Segal & Stewart, 1996), particularly if they suffer from symptoms of PTSD or other trauma-related disorder

(Cisler et al., 2011; Najavits, 2002; Ouimette, Moos, & Brown, 2003). As might be assumed based on its functional similarity to DRBs and dissociation, problematic drug and alcohol use is more common among those with low emotional regulation capacities (Kelly & Bardo, 2016) and a history of insecure attachment (Schindler & Bröning, 2015).

Summary: The RA Model Revisited

Taken together, clinical experience and an extensive psychological literature suggest that a range of seemingly dissimilar behaviors, whether self-injury, compulsive gambling, food bingeing and purging, dissociation, or problematic substance use, share an important underlying role: They all allow continued functioning despite what otherwise might be overwhelming psychological distress. These coping mechanisms are centered primarily on avoidance, allowing the survivor of painful life experiences to numb, self-soothe, distract, or separate from emotional pain. At the same time, however, these strategies can block emotional processing of painful memories, lead to future distress through the suppression effect, and increase vulnerability to new dangers and additional victimization.

This conundrum sets the stage for the subsequent chapters of this book. DRBs are used to decrease distress in the face of intolerable emotional pain, yet they tend to both help and hurt, protect and endanger. In this context, many people have a difficult time giving up problematic behaviors that they see as effective survival strategies. Yet avoidance responses can interfere with the development of new insights, for example, that avoidance behaviors may not be as necessary as they appear, that they may be causing harm, and, ultimately, that there may be better ways to survive.

CHAPTER 3

Key Treatment Recommendations

The RA perspective suggests a number of interventions that have proven helpful for those struggling with DRBs, ranging from relational psychotherapy and titrated memory processing to mindfulness training and trigger management. Beyond these specific interventions, presented in Chapters 5–9, however, are a number of treatment recommendations that are broadly relevant to avoidance-related responses.

Decrease Danger and Harm

Although DRBs and other avoidance behaviors have adaptive functions, many of them are intrinsically risky. Purging, for example, is associated with cardiac issues and gastric rupture; self-injury can cause bodily disfigurement; compulsive sexual behaviors can lead to life-threatening diseases; suicide attempts, obviously, may result in death; and substance use is associated with a wide range of medical problems, as well as the possibility of accidental overdose. And the dangers are not all medical: Avoidance activities such as substance use or dissociation, by definition, decrease awareness, and thus reduce vigilance to potential threats, and DRBs such as compulsive sex and reactive aggression increase the likelihood of subsequent sexual or physical assaults.

Given these various risks, therapy with the DRB-involved client must, above all, maximize safety, both in the client's environment and in terms of her own self-endangering behavior. As noted below, however, it is important that the clinician not respond in a "heavy-handed" or controlling manner regarding self-endangerment, but rather in a way that communicates caring and concern and, whenever possible, ensures the client's continuing autonomy and self-determination.

This does not preclude the therapist's ethical (and sometimes legal) responsibility to intervene without the client's consent under certain circumstances, for example, when mandated reporting or involuntary hospitalization is required to keep the client or others safe, including when the client is a parent or caretaker and a child is in danger. Even in such cases, however, the clinician should try to honor as much client agency as possible, and to employ the minimal amount of external control necessary.

Focus on the Therapeutic Relationship

Except for the ongoing need to keep the client safe, perhaps the most important component of RA-oriented treatment is a positive, mutually engaged therapeutic alliance. The quality of the therapeutic relationship has been shown to be one of the best predictors of treatment outcome in general (Ardito & Rabellino, 2011; Martin, Garske, & Davis, 2000; Norcross, 2011), let alone in the treatment of DRBs and other avoidance responses (e.g., Bedics, Atkins, Harned, & Linehan, 2015; Cronin, Brand, & Mattanah, 2014), in which safety, trust, and connection are especially important. Because many DRBs arise from attachment- and abuse-related deprivation and danger, the therapeutic relationship is most helpful when it is characterized by the directly opposing qualities of safety, caring, dependability, boundary awareness, and attunement. As various writers have suggested (e.g., Alexander & French, 1946; Siegel & Solomon, 2013), these aspects of the therapy relationship can help to counter the client's underlying assumptions of unacceptability and unlovability, and offer direct evidence that others can be sources of safety and caring.

As discussed in Chapter 8, a positive therapeutic relationship also allows the client to process negative childhood-era memories. As attachment dynamics are activated by the client–therapist relationship (referred to in this book as *relational activation*), two things are likely to occur: (1) Early, largely nonverbal memories are triggered, appearing as negative perceptions, thoughts, and feelings, yet (2) there is no actual danger or rejection in the therapy room—in fact, there is therapeutic safety and caring. This repeated juxtaposition of (1) archaic expectations of danger and rejection with (2) their antithesis, can slowly extinguish the connection between triggering phenomena and subsequent emotional distress.

Such relational reworking can have lasting positive effects based on what researchers describe as *reconsolidation* (Tronson & Taylor, 2007): the recent discovery that activated trauma memories are temporarily malleable, during which time they can be updated with new information and altered emotional associations. When this revised memory is then reconsolidated into neural tissue, the new memory will contain the added information (e.g., that one is no longer in danger, and that one is cared for) and emotional tone (e.g., reduced anxiety), leading to less triggerable distress and less need for DRBs. This new perspective on the effects of relational counterconditioning and reconsolidation is more fully explored in Chapter 8.

Above and beyond memory processing effects, a positive, attuned therapeutic relationship allows the client to do the difficult work of therapy in a reliable and safe environment—one characterized by the therapist's unconditional positive regard, empathy, and emotional availability (e.g., Rogers, 1957). In fact, clinical experience suggests that often it is only when the client is able to experience a "secure base" (Bowlby, 1988) and the stress-buffering effects of a sustained, positive therapeutic relationship that she can begin to approach distress rather than avoiding it, explore memories and feelings despite their painful qualities, and reevaluate early attachment-related assumptions about self and others.

Practice Nonjudgment and Monitor Countertransference

Many of those involved in behaviors such as self-injury, compulsive sexual behavior, or bingeing and purging view themselves as unacceptable and shameful (e.g., Deliberto & Nock, 2008; Murray, Waller, & Legg, 2000). Part of this is because DRBs are generally seen by society as bad or sick, with the result that each instance of cutting, stealing, or bingeing, for example, offers another opportunity for the individual to accumulate feelings of shame, self-disgust, and helplessness. As well, the child maltreatment and/or insecure attachment experiences that typically underpin the client's DRBs usually carry with them their own assumptions and beliefs involving the inadequacy of self and the danger of others (e.g., Briere, 2002a).

In this context, a nonjudgmental therapeutic stance is obviously important. Yet, as a member of society, the clinician may have opinions on "bad" behavior and what should be done about it, perhaps especially if the client's DRBs include aggression, indiscriminate sexual behaviors, or other forms of social rule breaking. As well, therapists, almost by definition, are likely to experience the activation of their own unresolved histories or issues when treating survivors of trauma and/or attachment disturbance (Dalenberg, 2000; Elliott & Guy, 1993). For example, the sometimes uncertain pace of treatment, and the client's resistance to giving up DRBs that he associates with survival, may lead to countertransferential feelings of impatience or inadequacy, or even anger in the therapist. As Linehan (1993) notes more broadly, the latter response may be most intense when the client is communicating extreme suffering, yet does not appear to be improving (or may even be deteriorating) with treatment. Similarly, the client's use of self- or other-endangering DRBs may cause significant therapist stress based on fears of legal or professional liability. In some cases, the client's abandonment concerns and sensitivity to rejection may result in negative responses to the therapist, which in turn can trigger the clinician's own reactions to unfair judgment or criticism.

Although countertransference and related therapist responses are understandable, they can be, of course, antithetical to the needs of the DRB-involved client, whose difficulties may escalate in the face of judgment. Sometimes referred to as *counteractivation,* because it refers to triggering of the therapist's own childhood memories and schema by client behaviors (e.g., Briere & Lanktree, 2012; Briere & Scott, 2014), this form of countertransference is not intrinsically a pathological response. Instead, it reflects the reality that the therapist, too, can be triggered by what occurs in the session.

There are many avenues for therapists who wish to decrease the incursion of judgment and other negative activations in the therapeutic process. These include one's own therapy, good supervision or consultation, and even certain meditation practices (e.g., *metta*; Salzberg, 2002). Most immediately, however, clinicians who find themselves triggered into judgmental responses may gain from consideration of a central principle of the RA model.

Specifically, the RA model holds that DRBs and other forms of problem behavior are not freely chosen actions, but rather arise from triggered trauma- or attachment-related emotional states that are potentially overwhelming in the absence of sufficient emotional regulation. Although this perspective may not always be sufficient to sustain equanimity after particularly stressful interactions with DRB-involved clients, it may allow the therapist to see the reduced behavioral control available to the client when he is triggered and desperate (Briere, 2012). To the extent that the clinician can discern the lack of "fault" inherent in triggered responses, she may be able to switch the focus from the client's challenging behavior to the pain that underlies it. Notably, this does not mean that the therapist feels pity, but rather, compassion—appreciating the complexity of adversity and its effects on both client and therapist, with a desire to reduce the client's suffering from things well beyond his control. This may including reminding oneself that the client is doing the best that he can, given the hand he has been dealt in life.

It is not just negative counteractivation that can arise in work with DRB-involved clients. Equally importantly, the therapist and client may both be affected by the power of emotional material that emerges when a previously suppressing trauma survivor is able to truly "open up" in the context of a safe, supportive, and caring relationship. The client may feel that she has finally found someone who understands and is willing to connect in an authentic way. As well, her disclosures and expressions of heretofore unexpressed experience may be intense and reflect a desire for previously unexperienced, attachment-level closeness. When managed well, this client response can deepen therapy and allow access to less available relational schema and sometimes still-raw attachment or trauma memories. It can also be a source of legitimate fulfillment for the clinician, who is able to see the fruits of her time, investment, and skill.

At the same time, however, the intensity of some RA-focused sessions can activate unprocessed feelings and attachment schemas in the therapist, including needs to parent, rescue, befriend, protect, or even romanticize or sexualize the client. These impulses and activations obviously must not be acted upon, and should be processed with a consultant, supervisor, or one's own therapist. Most basically, as noted in Chapter 8, trauma processing requires *disparity*: a lack of agreement between what the client feels or expects based on the past, and what she experiences in the present. This especially involves safety, both physically, and from therapist behaviors that are self-focused rather than in the service of the client's recovery and growth. This includes not only any kind of sexual behavior but also any attempts to gratify the therapist's needs to be special, or to experience emotional intimacy. Because source attribution errors occur for clinicians as well as clients, it may sometimes be difficult for the therapist to discern the attachment- or trauma-related reasons for her positive feelings—especially since therapeutic compassion and caring are critical parts of effective RA-based treatment. For this reason, it is recommended that the clinician carefully inspect any strong positive feeling that arises in the context of therapy for the possibility that it is counteractivation rather than solely due to nonegocentric caring.

Counter Demoralization and Encourage Hope

Because sustained DRBs and substance use are only temporarily effective, and are often followed by more desperation and distress, those involved in such behaviors often become increasingly demoralized and hopeless over time (Najavits, 2002). Repetitive anonymous sex, self-cutting, bingeing and purging, and compulsive gambling, for example, often occur in secrecy because they are experienced as shameful, even though they transiently reduce other painful feelings. Over the longer term, chronic DRBs and substance abuse can lead to increased risk of assault, lost relationships, bankruptcy, medical or psychiatric hospitalizations, imprisonment, disease or disfigurement, and other adverse circumstances that reinforce shame, alienation, helplessness, and hopelessness. In fact, these experiences can lead to a downward spiral of intensifying distress and even greater reliance on avoidance behaviors, the end point of which is sometimes referred to as *hitting bottom* in 12-step program terminology.

The "bottom" for some DRB-involved people may be the streets. As noted by an RA-oriented psychiatrist who works with the homeless,

> Many of my patients on skid row have experienced early and adult-life traumatic events, and many have diminished emotional regulation capacities. Some of them have some ability to self-regulate, but even for those, it seems like the grind of the daily low-level distress mounts and mounts until, one day, they explode. Maybe they have aggressive encounters, they relapse after a good period of sobriety, they engage in a sexual encounter in which they know they shouldn't engage, they max out their credit card, or spend all of their social security check. When they engage in these DRBs, they often suffer greatly as a result. Consequences can include eviction from housing, ejection from assistive programs, and loss of relationships. To complicate matters more, when DRBs include aggression in clinical office settings, they may result in termination from medical and mental health treatment settings, further leading to isolation and poor access to care. (John Jimenez, personal communication, February 18, 2018)

Although much of this book is concerned with clinical strategies to assist the DRB-involved client, and thus to reverse or forestall this spiral, it is often helpful at the outset to adopt a perspective on the client and his difficulties that is hopeful and "idealistic" (Najavits, 2002). *Idealism* in this context does not mean unrealistic expectations, but rather an overall philosophy that encourages the client to aspire to a more positive future and to access a sense of hope and self-efficacy. Although the therapist should not discount the sometimes incredible suffering that the client has experienced, it is often helpful to suggest that her continued survival and willingness to attend and stay in treatment—as well as any signs of improvement, no matter how small—reveals strength, adaptability, progress, and hope for a better future.

This hopefulness can be conveyed in several ways. The client can be encouraged to explore the actual functions of his DRBs, so that they can be reframed not as immoral or pathological behaviors but rather as coping responses to early life adversities. As the "badness" of substance use or compulsive stealing is reinterpreted and detoxified, for example, the client may be more able to identify self-characteristics such as courage, mental toughness, concern for the welfare of others, and even posttraumatic growth (Tedeshi & Calhoun, 2004)—phenomena that were present but hidden by the client's negative self-perceptions. For example, the homeless person who sees herself as manipulative, untrustworthy, and a "whore," based on what she has to do to deaden pain and increase her prospects for survival, may come to see herself in a more positive light as she considers, with the therapist's help, the paradoxically life-affirming reasons she engages in DRBs and/or substance use. At the same time, the clinician may work with the client to consider things she does that are idealistic in nature, such as daydreaming about a successful and happy future, trying to get a job, attempting to reduce or stop using a DRB or substance (even if unsuccessful), creating art, writing in a journal, or providing advice or sharing food with someone else on the streets.

Initially, the client may have difficulty identifying behaviors that are hopeful or idealistic, as opposed to the easy enumeration of her failures and unacceptable actions. Yet the therapist's steadfast attempts to reframe and redirect the client's view of her "bad" behavior can shift the client's perspective toward hopefulness and self-validation.

Avoid Authoritarian or Confrontational Behaviors

As noted earlier, given the client's sometimes precarious safety and continued self-endangerment, it can be difficult for the therapist not to over-exert control, or respond in ways that may occasionally seem demanding or even parental. Although some therapist responses may reflect counter-activation, it is also true that the clinician has some responsibility to try to keep the client safe, and to be unequivocal when a given response or plan is especially harmful to self or dangerous to others. The client may "pull" for this as well by seeking directive therapist behavior, clear instructions, and freedom from ambiguity, based on his perceived need for a strong and protective attachment figure.

This balance between avoiding potentially authoritarian behaviors, yet striving to increase client safety, can be a significant challenge in work with survivors of child abuse or disrupted attachment. The dangers here are several. The therapist who frequently confronts or challenges clients regarding their maladaptive or unsafe behavior runs the risk of appearing judgmental or rejecting, which may backfire by increasing their clients' guilt and shame, and inadvertently engendering further avoidance behaviors. Overly controlling therapist behaviors, whatever their etiology, also may undermine the client's sense of self-determination and autonomy, and reinforce abuse-related expectations of the therapist as a dominant person who must be appeased or, alternatively, rebelled against (Briere & Lanktree, 2012). In fact, for clients with attachment-level memories of rejection and maltreatment, controlling or authoritarian therapist behaviors may trigger anger and fear, challenge the therapeutic relationship and motivate even more extreme DRBs.

Although it may be a challenging task for the concerned (and perhaps activated) therapist, clinical experience suggests that the appropriate response to client DRBs is continued positive regard, compassion without pity, and a problem-solving and hopeful (rather than catastrophizing) perspective. In fact, the therapist can respond to a new DRB not as a failure of will or impulse control but rather as an opportunity for both the therapist and client to learn more about the client's triggers and what needs to be done in order to reduce the likelihood or intensity of future DRBs.

Provide Explicit Psychoeducation on DRBs and Childhood Adversity

One complexity associated with an RA perspective is described by Linehan (1993), involving the tension between two somewhat opposing ideas: (1) Triggered behaviors are rarely within the client's complete control, yet (2) it is important that the client strive for self-efficacy and self-determination. Like DBT, RA-oriented therapy tends to embrace both of these positions, generally by not only acknowledging the power of triggered trauma reactions, which are not the client's "fault," but also stressing that, through active participation in therapy, the client can gain increasing freedom from her childhood and greater control over her behavior and future well-being.

In many cases, the first step to this increased self-determinism is the client's greater understanding of what happened to him in the past, and how it manifests itself in the present. This is facilitated by discussions regarding the role of childhood insecure attachment and trauma in the genesis of DRBs, as well as the general principles of reactive avoidance. The goal is not for clients to find an "excuse" for their behavior, but rather to understand the psychological basis for their otherwise illogical, if not seemingly pathological, responses.

As noted at various points in this book, this growing awareness can counter inappropriate self-blame and shame, and provide clients with insights into the mechanics of triggers, overwhelming states, and DRBs, so that they can begin to change what happens to them in life. For example, a client may come to understand that she cuts herself to avoid early sexual abuse-related distress, or she engages in compulsive sexual behavior to fill the emptiness and isolation associated with early parental neglect. Once the connection between triggers, negative thoughts and feelings, emotional dysregulation, and DRBs become more clear, the client may be motivated to engage in treatment modalities that otherwise would not make as much sense, such as trigger management, therapeutic exposure to trauma memories, relational processing of attachment disturbance, and mindfulness.

It is usually important that clients also receive psychoeducation on the potential negative side effects of whatever DRBs or avoidance strategies they employ. This must be done in a nonjudgmental, nonlecturing manner, and should not involve scare tactics. Instead, the goal is for the clinician, in a compassionate way, to make sure that the client fully understands the sometimes very negative effects of his distress reduction activities. This may require considerable skill on the part of the therapist, since the goal is for the client to know about what she is risking, yet not be shamed, excessively frightened, or pathologized. In other words, the therapist is, in some ways, providing the client with "informed consent" regarding the impacts of her DRBs—not to frighten her into stopping the behavior per se, but to help her to be fully cognizant of the trade-offs involved.

Focus on Emotional Regulation

As noted earlier, childhood maltreatment tends to interfere with the development of emotional regulation capacities, perhaps especially if it disrupts parent–child attachment or dysregulates early neurobiology. As we will see in later chapters, the role of insufficient emotional regulation in the development of DRBs points to a clear clinical target: If we can increase the client's ability to internally "handle" negative emotional states, we can decrease her need for external avoidance strategies, including DRBs. In fact, most modern therapies for people engaged in problematic avoidance, whether DRBs, suicidality, dissociation, or problematic substance use, emphasize the importance of teaching emotional regulation skills (e.g., Blaustein & Kinniburgh, 2010; Cloitre, Cohen, & Koenen, 2006; Habib, Labruna, & Newman, 2013; Miller, Rathus, & Linehan, 2007).

Beyond the logical value of teaching emotional regulation to those involved in emotional avoidance, it is often important to strengthen the client's emotional capacities before major trauma or attachment memories can be directly processed during treatment (Courtois, Ford, & Cloitre, 2009; Herman, 1992b). This is because those involved in DRBs lack, almost by definition, sufficient ability to regulate triggered distress and are therefore at greater risk of being overwhelmed when treatment includes extended exposure to painful memories. In this sense, the presence of one or more DRBs can be seen as a marker for the likelihood that activated attachment or trauma memories may produce powerful negative emotions—reactions that may potentially overwhelm some clients during therapy.

Titrate Exposure and Activation

Despite these concerns, rarely is it necessary to entirely eschew memory processing when treating those with limited emotional regulation skills. It is more important that, at any given point, the client's activation–regulation balance is such that exposure to traumatic memory does not exceed his current emotional regulation capacities—a process sometimes referred to as *titrated exposure* or *working within the therapeutic window* (e.g., Briere, 1989; Briere & Scott, 2014). As noted in Chapter 8, the exact balance between how much trauma processing can safely occur versus how much emotional skills development needs to be in place is usually contingent on the severity of the client's triggered trauma or attachment memories and her immediate emotional regulation capacity. Nevertheless, in cases in which avoidance responses such as DRBs or problematic substance use are prominent, early treatment tends to focus considerably more on emotional regulation than on trauma or attachment processing, at least until emotional capacities are sufficiently developed. In less common cases (i.e., when DRBs are present but not accompanied by significant emotional dysregulation), therapeutic window issues may be less relevant, and exposure may require less titration.

Appendix 6 provides an In-Session Emotional Regulation and Activation Scale (ERAS), which the therapist uses to estimate the client's (1) current capacity to down-regulate distress without being overwhelmed, and (2) current level of activatable distress, and, thus, his overall activation–regulation balance. Although these ratings are based on subjective evaluations, they can help the therapist to consider how much trauma processing is possible without exceeding the therapeutic window.

Process Implicit Memories, as Well as Explicit Ones

Most trauma-related interventions focus on processing specific painful events from the past, generally by asking the client to remember and talk about the trauma in detail. As discussed in Chapter 8, repeated nonoverwhelming exposure to traumatic memories during therapy allows the associated negative emotions and thoughts to be reexperienced in a safe environment, and eventually extinguish.

However, memories that we can talk about are, by definition, autobiographical or explicit ones, involving a verbally mediated representation of what happened in the past. In contrast, there is a second memory type, sometimes described as sensory–emotional or implicit. One of the differences between these two systems is that explicit memories (the what, when, where of remembered events) are mostly encoded when a person's language capacities are relatively developed, whereas in the early, nonverbal years of life—when attachment processes are most active—only implicit memories (i.e., feelings, sensations, and nonverbal thoughts) are possible (Siegel, 2012). This has significant implications for "remembering": Explicit memories can usually be voluntarily recalled as such. Implicit memories, on the other hand, can only be triggered, at which point they are typically relived as current experiences, rather than past events.

This differentiation is critical to the way in which attachment problems are manifest in the adolescent or adult. As we see in Chapter 8, implicit memories of attachment insecurity, breaches, or losses cannot be recalled verbally, but they can be triggered into awareness by reminiscent stimuli in the current environment. For example, a person who experienced neglect or loss in the early years of life (let's call him Raymond) would not be able to explicitly recall much or anything from that time period, but still might be easily triggered into childhood-era feelings of abandonment or rejection by current relational stimuli.

The implications of implicit attachment encoding are highly relevant to the treatment of DRBs. If the memories underlying DRBs were largely explicit, traditional trauma processing through verbally mediated exposure therapy would likely be helpful. But early attachment memories are mostly implicit—they cannot be talked about, only triggered. And if they cannot be verbalized, they cannot be processed through classic exposure procedures.

This last treatment principle has to do with this conundrum. In order to assist Raymond in processing attachment-era distress, therapy must include ways to address implicit, as well as explicit, childhood memories. Fortunately, relational and attachment-oriented psychotherapists have long been working with this problem. What they have discovered and is only now receiving empirical support (see, e.g., Courtois & Ford, 2015), is that the therapeutic relationship can be a form of nonverbal, implicit, attachment-focused exposure therapy (Briere & Scott, 2014). Instead of asking the client to talk about what he cannot verbally recall, this form of exposure occurs when aspects of the therapeutic process trigger nonverbal memories of earlier relationships, especially those of childhood.

As more fully described in Chapter 8, when implicitly encoded, painful attachment-related thoughts and feelings (e.g., fear, anger, expectations of abandonment) are triggered in a positive therapeutic relationship, distress is activated but not reinforced. In the Raymond example, regular contact with a caring attachment figure (his therapist) will likely trigger attachment-era distress and early relational expectations, which will not be reinforced in the absence of current danger, rejection, or neglect; in fact they will be contradicted by experiences of safety and acceptance. Such "corrective emotional experiences" (Alexander & French, 1946), over time, can reduce the extent to which Raymond will be triggered into negative states by relational stimuli.

Adjust Treatment According to Severity and Presence of Broader Personality Disturbance

As noted in Chapter 1, most individuals who engage in DRBs are unlikely to meet criteria for BPD; in fact, DRBs are far more prevalent in clinical populations than is BPD. As a result, RA-focused treatment specifically targets the trauma and attachment memories, emotional dysregulation, and trigger dynamics often associated with DRBs, and devotes less attention to BPD domains such as emptiness, idealization–devaluation, severe identity disturbance, boundary issues, and splitting.

When these additional issues are present, however, and/or DRBs are so extreme that they represent immediate danger to the client, the RA treatment described in this book may be augmented with additional intervention components, including inpatient psychiatric hospitalization or residential treatment, psychopharmacology, and other treatments that more specifically target BPD symptoms or problems. In some cases, when the criteria for BPD are obviously present and especially relevant, the clinician may choose to integrate the trigger management and memory processing aspects of RA into a comprehensive DBT approach. Just as cognitive-behavioral therapy (CBT) for trauma has recently been combined with DBT to address sexual abuse-related PTSD in residential settings (e.g., Steil, Dyer, Priebe, Kleindienst, & Bohus, 2011), there is no obvious reason why DBT cannot be combined with RA interventions, perhaps especially during the "Stage 2" (Linehan, 1993) phase of treatment. Similarly, those diagnosed with BPD might gain from combining RA-focused treatment with mentalization-based therapy (MBT; Bateman & Fonagy, 2010), another validated treatment for BPD. As noted earlier, especially in the case of BPD in which there are persistent and dangerous DRBs, one treatment approach definitely may not fit all clinical presentations, and the client may be best served by augmenting or adjusting treatment to her specific needs and issues.

CHAPTER 4

Assessing Distress Reduction Behaviors in Context

As described in Chapters 1 and 2, the cascade of events and processes that lead to reactive avoidance (RA), including distress reduction behaviors (DRBs), is often quite complex, involving

- Early child maltreatment and loss
- Parental disattunement and disengagement
- Painful trauma and attachment memories, implicit and explicit
- Attachment disturbance, including altered assumptions about self and others
- Emotional regulation difficulties
- Current triggered distress, often in the context of some combination of immediate danger, stress, social marginalization, and/or continuing maltreatment.

To add to the complexity, each of these events and processes varies from one client to another, and contributes in different ways to RA. One person, for example, may suffer from profound neglect early in life, whereas another may be more affected by childhood sexual abuse experiences or later traumas. One person may develop an insecure attachment pattern characterized by avoidance of relationships and emotions, whereas another may become preoccupied with fears of abandonment and respond with neediness and emotional intensity. Some clients may be relatively adept at regulating the emotional effects of their early life experiences, whereas others may be plagued by overwhelming, uncontrollable emotions.

Even these adversity-related emotional states can be complex: In one person, emptiness, anger, guilt, or shame may be prominent, whereas posttraumatic stress, anxiety, and depression may be more relevant for a different person, and yet another may be especially prone to unwanted numbing, disconnection, and dissociation.

In combination with biological, cultural, and/or familial factors, these different antecedents and effects may require different coping responses, leading to different DRBs—for example, self-injury rather than compulsive sexual behavior. Finally, different DRBs may have different side effects, some of which may be more problematic or dangerous than others.

Without these distinctions, all forms of reactive avoidance and their underlying functions might be seen as equivalent (e.g., generic "acting out," impulsivity, or "borderline behavior"), resulting in a one-size-fits-all approach to intervention. In reality, treatment may vary considerably from one avoidance response to another, depending on the underlying etiology and the specific functions a given behavior serves. In one case, the primary interventions may be relational processing of implicit attachment memories and increasing the client's emotional regulation skills. In another therapeutic exposure, mindfulness training, and trigger management may be more relevant. In a third, treatment may especially target dissociative symptoms or intrusive negative thoughts. Since the details associated with a specific avoidance response matter in terms of which treatment components are used, this chapter outlines the primary domains that require assessment in DRB-focused therapy.

Immediate Danger or Risks

As noted earlier, avoidance behaviors, although immediately reinforcing, are associated with problems and risks that must be evaluated at the onset of therapy and regularly thereafter, in order to keep the client as safe as possible. Generally, these side effects are as follows, although additional unlisted problems or risks may also accrue (American Psychiatric Association, 2000; Fong, 2006; Grant et al., 2010; Rushing, Jones, & Carney, 2003; Walsh, 2014):

- *Self-injury:* inadvertent severe injury; life threat; disfiguration; infection; scars.
- *Triggered suicidal behavior:* life threat; postattempt physical or cognitive disability, disfigurement.
- *Compulsive sexual behavior:* sexually transmitted infections; risk of assault; relational losses; incarceration after soliciting sex; occupational and social losses associated with inappropriate sexual behaviors.
- *Bingeing and purging:* electrolyte imbalance; nutritional deficiencies; seizures; cardiac problems; esophageal lesions; gastric rupture; dental erosion; obesity-related medical problems.

- *Compulsive gambling:* bankruptcy, extreme debt and other negative financial outcomes; relational losses; incarceration associated with fraud or forgery.
- *Compulsive stealing:* incarceration; criminal record; loss of reputation.
- *Reactive aggression:* physical assaults and injuries; life threat; incarceration; relational losses.
- *Compulsive skin picking, hair pulling:* infection; disfigurement.
- *Fire setting:* inadvertent burns; incarceration.
- *Compulsive Internet use:* social and occupation problems; carpal tunnel syndrome; impaired vision, financial problems; identity theft.

Whatever DRBs a client employs, the therapist should evaluate for all relevant outcomes and be prepared to intervene as needed. In some cases, of course, continuing DRBs mean ongoing endangerment and distress, and the clinician may have only partial success in reducing the associated health or social effects. Nevertheless, client safety should be the therapist's first concern.

Psychological Comorbidities

Also important are psychological problems or disorders that co-occur with a given DRB, since comorbidities are quite common among those involved in RA (American Psychiatric Association, 2013; Grant et al., 2010), and may need to be treated before or during DRB-related therapy. Among the psychological difficulties experienced by at least some clients are

- Other DRBs
- Suicidality
- Excessive or otherwise problematic substance use
- Posttraumatic stress
- Depression
- Severe anxiety
- Attachment insecurity
- Relational disturbance
- Somatization or somatoform disorders
- Obsessive–compulsive symptoms or disorder
- Dissociative symptoms or disorders
- Personality disorders
- Hypomania associated with bipolar affective disorder
- Psychosis

Suicidality

Of these outcomes, one of the most concerning is the increased likelihood of suicide. This risk is highest among those who have already exhibited suicidal behavior (Bostwick, Pabbati, Geske, & McKean, 2016), including triggered suicidality. Any suicide attempt (regardless of how serious it is judged to be) statistically increases the likelihood of another one, and life threat may occur to the extent that the individual's distress escalates over time, or a lethal attempt occurs by accident. In the latter case, for example, the client may intend to engage in a sublethal overdose, in order to express and externalize overwhelming feelings of anger or self-disgust, but miscalculate the dosage. Or the client might intend to cut his wrist deeply enough to feel pain, but accidentally sever a major blood vessel. For such reasons, it is a truism in the suicide prevention field that any suicide attempt, even those thought to be gestures, must be taken seriously.

Also at higher risk of suicide are those involved in self-injury, as noted earlier, even though such behaviors often reflects a desire to survive—rather than be overwhelmed by—powerful negative states. In some cases, what appear to be self-injurious DRBs are actually sublethal suicide attempts. For example, superficial cutting can be a "dry run" to determine whether the pain associated with a more lethal laceration is tolerable. In others, when self-injury is distress reducing, and yet suicide attempts also occur, other scenarios are possible:

- Both activities serve ultimately nonlethal functions (e.g., communication of distress or proximity seeking); thus, one does not negate the other.
- Emotional distress waxes and wanes over time, so that self-injury may be sufficient in one instance, but suicidal behavior may seem necessary on another occasion, when triggered states are more severe.
- Self-injury is invoked initially, but it is insufficient to reduce emotional pain to tolerable levels, and suicide becomes the final avoidance strategy.

Because suicide attempts are themselves avoidance behaviors, it is not surprising that they can occur in the context of other DRBs, such as bingeing and purging (Bodell, Joiner, & Keel, 2011), risky sexual behavior (Houck et al., 2008), triggered aggression (Gvion & Apter, 2011), and compulsive gambling (Newman & Thompson, 2003), as well as substance use (Harned, Najavits, & Weiss, 2006). Beyond their shared underlying motivations, many DRBs have shame as a side effect, and shame can be a powerful contributor to suicidal behavior (Leshner, 1997).

Given the relative frequency of suicidal thoughts or behaviors among those engaged in DRBs, it is generally recommended that clinician assess for suicidal ideation, intent, plans, means, and recent attempts on a regular basis when working with DRB-involved clients. In fact, it may be necessary to ask about suicidal ideations and behavior at the onset of treatment, and to follow up with additional inquiries throughout therapy. Although this may seem tedious or, alternatively, catastrophizing, the clinician's intention to do regular suicidality assessment can be introduced to the client at the beginning of treatment, so that its repeated occurrence is not overinterpreted or seen as unduly pathologizing. In introducing the idea of regular suicidality checks, the clinician reinforces how seriously she takes the client's well-being, and how dangerous certain DRBs can be, irrespective of their functional value to the client.

The specific extent of suicide assessment necessary will depend on the client's recent history of attempts, any comorbidities that are present (e.g., reduced emotional regulation capacity, depression, posttraumatic hyperarousal, dissociation, psychosis), whether he reports suicidal ideations, whether DRBs are becoming more intense or frequent of late, the current level of stress or adversity in his environment, and the extent of support from friends, family, and others. Several potentially useful psychological tests are presented below, although the reader should keep in mind that such measures do not always discriminate those who go on to attempt suicide from those who do not—they are more probabilistic than definitive (Fowler, 2012). Often, the best approach is initially to administer psychological testing that includes suicidality, then to follow up with gentle, nonpathologizing, but specific questions during intake and, as needed, in subsequent therapy sessions. If these informal questions indicate potential acute suicidality, more intensive testing and evaluation is then indicated. See books by Bongar and Sullivan (2013), Simon and Hales (2012), and Maris, Berman, Maltsberger, and Yufit (1992) for guidance on developing an overall approach to evaluating potential client suicidality, and Linehan's (1993) strategies for assessing and addressing suicidal behavior.

Assessment Tools

In many cases, the evaluation of DRB comorbidities is relatively straightforward, because the client is able to directly report, or clearly exhibits, problematic mood states, behaviors, or disorders. In others, however, the individual may be in denial about existing problems or symptoms, or may hide them from the clinician. In some cases, avoidance strategies are so successful that they conceal evidence of their own existence. For example, a client using denial or dissociation may not "know" that she is doing so, and the person engaging in indiscriminate sex to distract from, ironically, intimacy fears, may be superficially unaware that he is afraid of close connections.

Beyond report or awareness problems, the list of potential comorbidities is sufficiently long that some may not necessarily be considered by the clinician or disclosed by the client. In fact, research suggests that the typical unstructured clinical interview tends to overlook traumas and symptoms (e.g., Zimmerman & Matia, 1999) that are nevertheless relevant to the client's current situation.

For these reasons, when possible, it is recommended that those with significant DRB involvement be administered normed psychological tests or validated diagnostic interviews, either by the clinician if she is licensed to do so, or through referral to a psychologist. These not only include trauma exposure, attachment security, comorbid symptomatology, and types and functions of DRBs, but also social support, since this variable appears to have a significant impact on resilience to the effects of attachment- and trauma-related adversity (Weiss, Garvert, Cloitre, 2015; Kaniasty, 2005).

Presented below is a brief list of psychological tests and interviews that are directly relevant to the assessment of DRB-related issues. This is a small subset of potential measures, however; the clinician or consultant may find others that are even more useful.

- Broadband/generic assessment of symptomatology
  - Psychological Assessment Inventory (PAI; Morey, 1991)
  - Minnesota Multiphasic Personality Inventory–2 (MMPI-2; Butcher, Dahlstrom, Graham, Tellegen, & Kaemmer, 1989)—including the content scales [Butcher, Graham, Williams, & Ben-Porath, 1990] and the Restructured Form [Greene, 2010])
  - Minnesota Multiphasic Personality Inventory–Adolescent (MMPI-A; Butcher et al., 1992)
  - Symptom Checklist-90–Revised (SCL-90-R; Derogatis, 1983)
- Specific assessment of PTSD, dissociation disorder, and BPD
  - Clinician-Administered PTSD Scale for DSM-5 (CAPS-5; Weathers et al., 2018)
  - Posttraumatic Stress Diagnostic Scale (PDS; Foa, 1995)
  - Detailed Assessment of Posttraumatic Stress (DAPS; Briere, 2001)[1]
  - Dissociative Experiences Scale (DES; Bernstein & Putnam, 1986)
  - Multiscale Dissociation Inventory (MDI; Briere, 2002b)

---

[1] *Potential conflict of interest note:* The DAPS, MDI, TSI-2, TSCC, and IASC, listed in this section, were written by the author who receives royalties from Psychological Assessment Resources.

- o Zanarini Rating Scale for Borderline Personality Disorder (ZAN-BPD; Zanarini, Weingeroff, Frankenburg, & Fitzmaurice, 2015)
- Broadband assessment of complex posttraumatic outcomes
  - o Structured Interview for Disorders of Extreme Stress (SIDES; Pelcovitz et al., 1997)
  - o Trauma Symptom Inventory–2 (TSI-2; Briere, 2011)
  - o Trauma Symptom Checklist for Children (TSCC—includes adolescents up to 17 years old; Briere, 1996).
- Specific assessment of attachment- and emotional regulation-related symptoms
  - o Trauma and Attachment Belief Scale (TABS; Pearlman, 2003)
  - o Inventory of Altered Self Capacities (IASC; Briere, 2000)
  - o Insecure Attachment and Impaired Self-Reference scales of the TSI-2
  - o Experiences in Close Relationships—Revised (ECR-R; Fraley, Waller, & Brennan, 2000)
- Suicide assessment
  - o Beck Hopelessness Scale (Beck, Kovacs, & Weissman, 1975)
  - o Scale for Suicide Ideation (Beck, Kovacs, & Weissman, 1979)
  - o Adult Suicidal Ideation Questionnaire (Reynolds, 1991)
  - o Collaborative Assessment and Management of Suicidality, 2nd Edition (CAMS; Jobes, 2016)
- Social support
  - o Multidimensional Scale of Perceived Social Support (Zimet, Dahlem, Zimet, & Farley, 1988).
  - o Duke–UNC Functional Social Support Questionnaire (DUFSS; Broadhead, Gehlbach, deGruy, & Kaplan, 1988).
- Assessment of DRBs
  - o Self-injury
    - Functional Assessment of Self-Mutilation (FASM; Lloyd, Kelley, & Hope, 1997)
    - Deliberate Self-Harm Inventory (DSHI; Gratz, 2001)
  - o Risky or compulsive sexual behavior
    - Compulsive Sexual Behavior Inventory (CSBI; Miner, Coleman, Center, Ross, & Rosser, 2007)
    - Sexual Compulsivity Scale (SCS; Kalichman & Rompa, 2001)
    - Dysfunctional Sexual Behavior subscale of the TSI-2
  - o Bingeing/purging
    - Binge Eating Scale (BES; Gormally, Black, Daston, & Rardin, 1982)
    - Eating Disorder Examination Questionnaire (EDE-Q; Fairburn & Beglin, 1994)

○ Aggression
  ▪ Aggression Questionnaire (AQ; Buss & Warren, 2000)
  ▪ State–Trait Anger Expression Inventory–2 (STAXI-2; Spielberger, 1999)
○ Problem gambling
  ▪ Brief Biosocial Gambling Screen (BBGS; Gebauer, LaBrie, & Shaffer, 2010)
  ▪ Problem Gambling Severity Index (PGSI; Holtgraves, 2009; for modified scoring, see Currie, Hodgins, & Casey, 2013)
○ Compulsive theft
  ▪ Kleptomania Symptom Assessment Scale (K-SAS; Grant & Kim, 2002)
  ▪ Structured Clinical Interview for Kleptomania (SCI-K; Grant, Kim, & McCabe, 2006)
○ Problematic Internet use
  ▪ Compulsive Internet Use Scale (CIUS; Meerkerk, Van Den Eijnden, Vermulst, & Garretsen, 2009)
  ▪ Internet Addiction Test (IAT; Young, 1998)
○ Compulsive buying
  ▪ Bergen Shopping Addiction Scale (BSAS; Andreassen et al., 2015)
  ▪ Compulsive Buying Scale (CBS; Valence, d'Astous, & Fortier, 1988)
○ Fire setting
  ▪ Four Factor Fire Scale (FFFS; Ó Ciardha et al., 2016)
○ Hair pulling and skin picking
  ▪ Massachusetts General Hospital Hairpulling Scale (MGH-HPS; Keuthen et al., 1995)
  ▪ Skin Picking Scale (SPS; Keuthen et al., 2001)
○ Generalized involvement in distress reduction behavior
  ▪ The Tension Reduction Behavior scale of the TSI-2

Assessing for Childhood Abuse, Neglect, and Attachment Disturbance

Because DRBs and other forms of RA generally arise from negative events in childhood—often abuse, neglect, or parental nonresponsiveness, then attachment disturbance—it is generally helpful to assess for these adverse experiences. Sometimes this can be determined merely by asking clients, in behavioral terms, whether they have experienced childhood sexual, physical, or psychological abuse, or psychological neglect, and, if so, when it occurred. Examples of interviews or self-report child maltreatment inventories that can be used to collect this information are the Adverse

Childhood Experiences measure (ACE; Felitti et al., 1998), the Childhood Trauma Questionnaire—Short Form (CTQ-SF; Bernstein et al., 2003), the Child Maltreatment Interview Schedule (Briere, 1992), and the Initial Trauma Review for Adolescents (ITR-A; Briere & Lanktree, 2012).

In other cases, however, self-reports do not provide the information needed, for example when the client is not willing to share it, or when the maltreatment occurred before the development of explicit, autobiographic memory and thus cannot be verbally reported (Briere & Hodges, 2010). In the former case, the client may be more forthcoming as the therapeutic relationship deepens and she comes to trust the clinician. In the latter, the therapist can ask whether relatives or others ever mentioned or described abuse or neglect in the client's history, or whether there is other documentation (e.g., child abuse reports, hospitalization records) indicating that maltreatment may have occurred. In some cases, a nonabusive parent or sibling may be a better informant than the client regarding his early history, and the client may allow the therapist to explore this avenue.

Similar constraints are present for assessing parent–child attachment quality, since the most critical attachment years are prior to the onset of verbal memory. There are multiple measures that attempt to evaluate attachment security (e.g., the Experiences in Close Relationships questionnaire [ECR; Brennan, Clark, & Shaver, 1998], the Relationship Questionnaire [RQ; Bartholomew & Horowitz, 1991], and the attachment subscales of the TSI-2); unfortunately, they do so indirectly, asking people to report problems in their current close or intimate relationships that have been associated with early attachment difficulties. An alternative to this approach, the Disorganized Response Scale (DRS; Briere et al., 2018), evaluates disorganized attachment based on self-reports of dysregulated attachment behavior. This is a new measure, however, and is not yet standardized or normed.

Even in the absence of information in this area, the client and therapist still may be able to reconstruct some of what may have been the client's earlier experiences. For example, if the client recalls emotional or physical abuse at 5 or 6 years of age, it may be possible to hypothesize (but not guarantee) earlier maltreatment as well. Similarly, although the client will not be able to report on attachment experiences in the first years of life, she may be able to describe later maternal or paternal coldness, nonresponsiveness, rejection, fearfulness, frightening behavior, abandonment, problematic substance use, dissociation, depression, or emotional lability, all of which are associated with insecure attachment in children (e.g., Bowlby, 1969, 1988; Sroufe, Egeland, Carlson, & Collins, 2005; van IJzendoorn, 1995). Especially when these conjectures match the client's current clinical presentation (e.g., an insecure attachment style or hypersensitivity to authority, intimate relationships, and/or abandonment), a working therapeutic hypothesis may be formed about the client's early years, albeit one that is tentative and not assumed to be necessarily accurate. Importantly, the therapist should never assert that abuse or neglect has definitely occurred in such instances, since such insistence may produce memory errors in susceptible individuals (Lindsay & Briere, 1997).

RA Model Measures[2]

DRB Types and Characteristics

Once the antecedents to, and comorbidities of, behavioral avoidance have been considered, the next step is usually to determine what DRBs the client currently employs, as well as those she has used in the past. Appendix 2 contains a checklist (the Review of Distress Reduction Behaviors) that the therapist can include in the intake or subsequent interview. When completed, it provides information on all major types of DRBs, past and present, how often they are currently used, and when they began.

Triggers

As noted, DRBs usually occur after the individual has encountered a trigger in her current relational environment. Generally, a *trigger* can be defined as any stimulus that is sufficiently reminiscent of a past event or process that it activates implicit or explicit memories in the present. Many triggers of DRBs are interpersonal, for example, perceived rejection, abandonment, criticism, boundary violations, yelling, or maltreatment, although others may be noninterpersonal, such as certain sounds, smells, and tastes. Included in Appendix 3 is a Trigger Review, in which the client explores ways in which he has been triggered in the past, and what feelings, sensations, and thoughts tend to occur after he is triggered.

As well, a Triggers-to-Memories Worksheet can be found in Appendix 5. This form is more of a treatment tool than an assessment device per se, since it is used to assist the client in identifying and understanding the actual trauma-related etiologies of specific triggers. Use of this worksheet is discussed in Chapter 9.

Functions Served by DRBs

Finally, Appendix 4 contains a Functions of Distress Reduction Behaviors checklist, which clients complete separately for each type of DRB that they have employed. For example, a client involved in compulsive sexual

---

[2]All RA model measures are available to purchasers of this book (see the box at the end of the table of contents).

behavior might indicate that sexual DRBs distract from upsetting memories, soothe triggered distress, and lessen feelings of emptiness. Administration of this checklist may be an important initial part of treatment, since it indicates the actual reasons why any given DRB is being used and potentially highlights the best targets for treatment. For example, if the client indicates that self-injury blocks memories, distracts from triggered angry feelings, and lessens dissociation, the most helpful interventions might include emotional processing of specific memories, learning self-calming or self-grounding skills so that dissociation is less likely, and problem solving what the client might do instead of self-injury that would still address her immediate needs.

CHAPTER 5

Safety, Stabilization, and Harm Reduction

Antoine is a 32-year-old man who has struggled with compulsive gambling and excessive drinking for a number of years. He reports having "hit bottom" 4 months ago, after losing his apartment over unpaid rent, a brief hospitalization for acute gastritis, and a breakup with his boyfriend of 2 years. He has recently experienced a resurgence of PTSD-like symptoms, primarily flashbacks and sleep disturbance, which he links to a history of child maltreatment.

Antoine began therapy 2 months ago, but has thus far been unable to talk about his current situation or childhood history to any meaningful extent. In response, his therapist is teaching him relaxation techniques, grounding, harm reduction approaches to his alcohol use, and ways to identify and address triggers in his environment that lead to urges to gamble. She anticipates that it may be a while before Antoine is able to talk about his situation and its antecedents in any detail, but notes that early stabilization efforts have decreased his overall stress and insomnia.

Many DRB-involved clients enter therapy in relative chaos. They are often, as Freud once noted, plagued by "reminiscences" (Gay, 1989, p. 71)—not only explicit memories of childhood maltreatment and later traumas but also implicit ones, appearing in the guise of unidentifiable fears of abandonment or violence, unexpected thoughts, urges to do things that do not make sense, and moments of self-hatred or disgust. Because these reactions are based largely on past events for which the client may have little explicit memory, their sudden appearance is often frightening and unexpected, and may appear contextually inappropriate or even bizarre to others.

These difficulties are, ironically, often exacerbated by the client's attempts to control or suppress them. As discussed, the client may respond with behaviors that are sufficiently dramatic, disruptive, or deadening, that they are effective even against overwhelming emotions and memories. Yet, ultimately, these behaviors fail: DRBs such as self-injury, bingeing and purging, or risky sexual behaviors appear to "work" over the subsequent minutes or hours, but their long-term effects are usually problematic, if not debilitating or life-threatening. And, as it turns out, they actually tend to increase, not decrease, distress over time.

Creating a Supportive and Collaborative Therapeutic Relationship

It is within this context, at whatever level of extremity, that the client appears in the therapist's office, clinic, or hospital. Because of early experiences, she is prone not only to relive dangerous or hurtful moments from the past but also to assume peril in the present and future. And many of the things that the client does to keep painful memories and emotions at bay can result in further suffering, danger, and loss.

> Erick, a 17-year-old man who is attempting to separate himself from a neighborhood gang, has reluctantly entered psychotherapy at the insistence of his probation officer. Immediately hypervigilant in the intake interview, he challenges the therapist on confidentiality issues, why she does this work, her assumptions about him as a person of a different ethnicity, gender, and socioeconomic status, and the likelihood that therapy will be of any use to him. Early in the session, Erick has a strong response to the clinician's implication that she, and the therapy, are trustworthy. Raising his voice, and using a sudden barrage of gang words and phrases, he expresses his disbelief that therapy can be a safe place, and that he would be valued there. At the same time, the therapist notices, but does not comment on, what appears to be a hint of tears in Erick's eyes.

Although a variety of ways in which the clinician can increase the client's overall level of safety are described in this chapter, few of these principles or interventions will be helpful unless a positive and manifestly safe therapeutic relationship can be developed. Yet this is sometimes easier said than done. One of the early casualties of childhood abuse and neglect can be the easy availability of hope and trust, and the capacity to see safety and positive regard when they are present. For many traumatized people, closeness implies danger, kindness is bait for entrapment, and awareness causes pain. In fact, the basic assumptions of therapy—that one should open oneself up to a seemingly powerful other, believe this person's assertion that she is kind and can be trusted, and give up one's avoidant defenses because feeling bad, ultimately, is good for one—may seem counterintuitive and perhaps even dangerous. And, in many cases, the client's defenses are more or less correct: He may not, in fact, be ready to engage what he tries to avoid. In the co-presence of high pain and low emotional tolerance, some level of avoidance may be continuously necessary for internal homeostasis. Because his self-protective stance can serve real, adaptive functions, it is not necessarily healthy or wise to disregard hard-earned experience and immediately trust someone just because he is supposed to do so.

This is the difficult path that the client and therapist must engage if treatment is to be helpful. The client has the perfect right and reasons not to trust or connect with the therapist, yet most significant trauma and attachment processing occurs within trust and connection. And the therapist must repeatedly demonstrate (not just say) that she is trustworthy and that the client is safe with her, even though it may initially be difficult for the client to believe or accept these facts in progress. In this context, the therapist must work especially hard to stay attuned, empathic, positive, and caring, and remind herself that the client is, in fact, a survivor—the very behaviors that may seem pathological, defensive, or primitive may have allowed him to make it to the therapist's office in the first place (Butler, 1989).

It is also important that the therapeutic relationship be collaborative rather than a context in which the therapist provides unidirectional input regarding what is wrong and how it can be corrected. The clinician's focus should be on:

- Discussing with the client her rights to boundaries, safety, dignity, self-determination, and even self-protectiveness in the session.
- Working with her to identify problem behaviors and their impacts.
- Figuring out with her what drives them.
- Determining, together, what might be helpful in response.
- And, finally, coming up with a treatment plan that the client finds meaningful and acceptable.

The critical notion here is that, to the extent possible, the client is the final arbiter regarding what he wants to address and how therapy might proceed. This approach empowers the client, as it encourages the development of self-entitlement and problem-solving skills rather than continued reliance on the therapist for solutions.

Immediate Environmental Safety and Stability

One of the most immediate sources of danger for those engaged in DRBs is continuing threat from the environment. As noted, many DRB-involved people suffer from childhood maltreatment and attachment disturbance, both of which are associated with what clinicians refer to as *revictimization*— the tendency for those who were maltreated in childhood to experience additional violence (not only physical and sexual assaults but also psychologically hurtful relationships) in adolescence and adulthood (e.g., Koenig, Doll, O'Leary & & Pequegnat, 2003; Godbout et al., 2017).

The revictimization literature (e.g., Duckworth & Follette, 2012; Messman & Long, 1996; Messman-Moore, Walsh, & DiLillo, 2010; Widom, Czaja, & Dutton, 2008) suggests that risk of additional trauma can arise from a variety of abuse-related phenomena, including the following:

- Substance use and dissociation, both of which can reduce vigilance to danger.
- Distorted perceptions of others (e.g., idealization) that interfere with awareness of danger cues.
- Low self-esteem and a diminished sense of entitlement to safety.
- Risky behaviors that increase the likelihood of additional assaults, such as less discriminant sexual partner selection.
- Cognitive accommodation to ongoing violence, such that later interpersonal danger is discounted or accepted as normal.
- Relational difficulties such as learned helplessness or passivity in the face of danger, as well as willingness to tolerate maltreatment in order to forestall abandonment.
- Socioeconomic stressors and discrimination, both of which increase the likelihood of child maltreatment and later exposure to community violence.

Because these various factors tend to persist over time, the clinician should not assume that clients' traumas and attachment problems reside solely in the past; they may continue to be at risk of physical or sexual assault, exploitation, and emotional maltreatment, let alone social marginalization or poverty. This ongoing potential means that assessment should not be limited to clients' current symptomatology and DRBs; it should also extend to their physical, interpersonal, and sociocultural safety.

In some cases, this will include evaluating the continuing impacts of early violence that have been triggered by recent threats to safety.

Sokha is a 67-year-old woman who was sexually assaulted and tortured by Cambodian soldiers in the 1970s. Although she immigrated to the United States in the 1980s, she continues to limit her activities and travels within a single-block radius in her small, Khmer-speaking community. Soon after encountering a stranger who appeared to be an ex-member of the regime that tortured her, Sokha was found in her bedroom closet, scratching on her arms, legs, and chest, and crying out as if she was being sexually assaulted. After unsuccessful attempts at treatment at a county community health center, she now attends an Asian-Pacific mental health center, where her history and responses are well understood by staff members, and where she is able to process her triggered responses and current fears in greater perceived safety.

Along with continued assessment, the therapist must be prepared to intervene in whatever way necessary to increase client safety, which includes being willing to be relatively directive (but not overcontrolling) when indicated. In some cases, this may involve giving explicit, but not dogmatic, advice; working with the client to access law enforcement when he is in danger; dealing with social services around issues of homelessness or poverty; or arranging a medical referral in case of serious illness. In other instances, the therapist might provide psychoeducation about needle exchange programs, safer sex practices, medical risks of various DRBs, the location of shelters or self-help groups, and/or training in non-abusive parenting practices.

Immediate safety also may be increased by working with the client to stabilize her interpersonal environment, address immediate mental health concerns, and reduce her overall level of stress. This may include referring the client for couple or family therapy when these systems contribute to the client's difficulties; encouraging a psychiatric evaluation for medications or hospitalization when suicidality, a mood disorder, severe posttraumatic stress, or psychosis interferes with adaptive functioning; and problem solving around ways the client can reduce the chaos, demands, and challenges of his personal, school, or work environment. As noted by Herman (1992b) and others (e.g., Cloitre, Koenen, Cohen, & Han, 2002), the client also may benefit from early interventions and exercises that increase her emotional regulation capacities. As discussed later in this chapter, as well as in Chapter 7, this may include learning relaxation, grounding, and meditation techniques, as well as strategies for "taking better care of yourself" or "improving the moment" (Linehan, 1993) in challenging interpersonal contexts or situations.

Safety from Self-Harm

Not entirely separate from immediate environmental dangers, DRBs are, almost by definition, inherently self-endangering. As described previously,

DRB risks can include disability, disease, incarceration, exposure to violence, and death. Although major reduction of DRBs can require significant time in treatment, there are usually things the client can do early in the therapy process to increase safety from self-harm. Described in Chapter 7 as *trigger management,* this includes the following:

- Reducing the frequency of triggering events.
- Lessening the destabilizing effects of triggered states.
- Reducing the immediate harm associated with DRBs.

Trigger Reduction

An important early step in stabilization, *trigger reduction* involves identifying triggers associated with the client's most problematic DRBs, then exploring ways in which these triggers can be rendered less powerful or avoided entirely.

In some cases, trigger reduction may be used as a temporary measure, especially when continuous trigger avoidance would be problematic or unwanted. For example:

- Someone who is easily triggered and overwhelmed in verbal disputes with a friend might decide in treatment to avoid arguments with this person for the time being, even though conflictual issues must be addressed at some point in the future.
- A person might find that certain sexual situations or stimuli trigger childhood sexual abuse memories, and therefore avoid those situations, so that a given DRB (e.g., subsequent bingeing or shame-related self-injury) is less likely. Over time, however, the person also might develop greater emotional regulation capacities and engage in memory processing of abuse memories, both of which might make future consensual sexual contact less activating and potentially more enjoyable (Bigras, Daspe, Godbout, Briere, & Sabourin, 2017).

In other cases, trigger avoidance may be a more permanent solution, either because avoidance of the trigger is a good idea in general, or because the triggering situation can be avoided without any obvious deleterious effects. For example:

- A person who finds him- or herself angry and prone to aggression when around inebriated people might discover that contact with drunken people triggers memories of abuse by an intoxicated caretaker, and resolve to avoid bars and, hence, triggered bar fights.

- Someone who is triggered into painful memories when watching violent movies might decide to permanently avoid such films as a way to terminate unwanted distress.

Although trigger avoidance is unlikely to address entirely the client's sense of chaos and unpredictable intrusions, it is often an early opportunity for the client to slowly "take charge" of his immediate experience and environment. In some cases, the decreased turmoil associated with limiting exposure to triggers may also demonstrate to the client that she is not helpless, and, in fact, is able to increase her emotional stability.

Reducing the Destabilizing Effects of Triggered States

Because it is not possible, or even adaptive, to avoid all triggers in one's environment, the goals of early treatment often include (1) proactively increasing resilience to activated distress, so that DRBs are less probable or less intense when triggering occurs, and (2) mitigating the effects of activated emotions and thoughts after they occur and before they motivate DRBs.

Intervention in triggered states often requires increasing the client's emotional regulation skills as a way to equilibrate her activation–regulation balance. The need to intervene in emotional dysregulation when addressing avoidance behaviors was most prominently introduced to clinicians by Marsha Linehan in 1993. Initially focused on treating women with chronic suicidal behavior, and then BPD, DBT has been shown to have efficacy for the various behaviors described in this book, primarily self-injury, suicidality, bingeing–purging, and substance abuse in the context of borderline personality (e.g., Kliem, Kröger, & Kosfelder, 2010; Safer, Telch, & Agras, 2001), although see Panos, Jackson, Hasan, and Panos (2013). Given the breadth of Linehan's contributions, a number of the emotional regulation interventions recommended in this chapter and elsewhere either directly reflect DBT principles and techniques, or were inspired by them.

Proactive Resilience

Many individuals heavily involved in DRBs or substance use neglect their physical health or suffer health problems, because their avoidance behaviors have secondary physical effects. As a result, they may have fewer internal resources available to deal with triggered distress, leading to more DRBs. Linehan (2014) specifically enumerates ways to increase resilience, as defined by her PLEASE acronym:

- Treat **P**hysical i**L**lness.
- Balance **E**ating.
- Avoid mood-**A**ltering drugs or alcohol.
- Balance **S**leep.
- **E**xercise.

Although increasing resilience—and thus decreasing emotional vulnerability—might seem like a relatively easy first step toward stabilization, in fact it may be difficult. For example, sleeping or eating well may be especially challenging for people who are homeless, experiencing ongoing danger, or suffering from PTSD or an eating disorder. Because drug or alcohol use is an avoidance strategy, it may be hard for the beleaguered person to lessen or give it up. Similarly, seeking medical assistance might seem like an easy action, but many of those who rely on avoidance behaviors also avoid medical checkups or seeking medical advice, lest the news be bad.

This does not mean that these activities are not an important component of early intervention, because they are often quite central to early stabilization. At the same time, however, the clinician should be prepared for potential roadblocks in this area, and must not engage in adversarial struggles with the client to "just" take better care of herself.

Beyond the development of internal resources, an additional approach to resiliency involves intentionally connecting with people with whom one can process, debrief, and recover from stressful situations. Not all traumatized or attachment-dysregulated people, let alone those involved in DRBs, can easily access others for support and nurturance, of course, and many may fear such connections because they are associated with previous maltreatment, rejection, or loss. Nevertheless, a support group, or even just a reliably caring and validating person (or sponsor), can be of substantial benefit to those who suffer from early trauma or attachment insecurity. In fact, social support is thought to be among the most powerful contributors to resilience among traumatized people (see Kaniasty, 2005, for a review).

For this reason, clinical intervention in this area often involves increased therapeutic attention to the client's experiences with friends, caretakers, or partners. For example, the clinician might help the client to work through interpersonal difficulties with others that might otherwise cause relational breaches, rather than just focusing on her history and internal experiences. In other instances, the therapist may gently suggest the client attend nonthreatening social events, or (subject to client agreement and comfort level) 12-step or support groups that are especially relevant to his history, circumstance, or DRBs.

Alternatively, when interpersonal support is difficult to find, too threatening, or insufficient, some traumatized or attachment-reactive individuals find that a pet, for example a dog or cat, can provide a sense of noncontingent love, acceptance, and relationship that might not otherwise be immediately available, or even tolerable. Although the literature on the specific helpfulness of animal assisted therapy is equivocal, albeit encouraging, studies suggest that living with a companion animal can be especially grounding and stabilizing for people struggling with chronic difficulties and/or perceived social unacceptability (e.g., Brooks, Rushton, Walker, Lovell, & Rogers, 2016; McConnell, Brown, Shoda, Stayton, & Martin, 2011).

Mitigating the Immediate Stressfulness of Triggered Thoughts, Emotions, and Memories

There are a number of trigger management activities that, if engaged in immediately following a triggering event, can reduce subsequent distress and therefore lessen the need for DRBs or other avoidance responses. They include the following.

Breath and Relaxation Training

Learning how to relax and slow one's breath can be of tremendous benefit when in a stressful situation, or immediately following triggered emotional reactions. Typically, the client practices focused breathing or other forms of relaxation across multiple sessions, as well as at home, then gradually learns to apply these skills at times of triggered distress. In some cases, this also involves mindfulness training, as described in Chapter 6. As the client is increasingly able to enter a more calm or relaxed state, despite, for example, activated fear or anger, the need for a DRB may decrease. Two breathing exercises are presented in Appendix 1, each of which can be practiced both in the therapist's office and later at home.

Importantly, the key issue is usually not the acquisition of relaxation or breath skills, but rather the client's increasing ability to apply these new abilities when experiencing painful memories or states. This capacity can be strengthened during specific moments in therapy, when the client—with the therapist's support—learns to apply mindful breathing or other relaxation exercises at times of upset or distress.

Grounding

Grounding usually involves learning to focus on the immediate external environment, and the current moment, as a way to pull attention away from escalating internal states associated with painful memories. Like relaxation training, this skill can be taught when the client experiences strong negative emotions in the session and, thus, is able to practice grounding at times of momentary destabilization. The client is typically asked to describe the surrounding room or environment in detail, to practice mindful breathing or a relaxation exercise, and to engage in positive self-talk, as described below. The clinician may quietly model grounding statements, noting, for example, that the client is safe in the *here* (in the room, in the session, with the therapist) and the *now* (not in the past, in danger, undergoing the trauma) (Briere & Scott, 2014). Although grounding is sometimes presented as an acute intervention for when clients are overwhelmed in treatment, it is even more helpful as a learned skill that can be applied outside of the session—especially when triggered emotions, thoughts, or memories occur.

Self-Soothing

Self-soothing can be defined as self-directed behaviors that increase feelings of well-being, calm, and self-care. The term *soothing* in this context usually refers to a central notion in attachment theory: that memories of loving physical contact, hugging, rocking, cuddling, and protective care by early attachment figures can be internalized by the individual, and later called upon as a form of emotional regulation in the face of stressful circumstances. Whether self-soothing always activates attachment-level phenomena is unknown. However, many survivors of childhood trauma report that engaging in activities that are explicitly self-nurturing and self-caring can diminish the emotional effects of triggered memories.

Some self-soothing behaviors, for example, thumb sucking, rocking, or cuddling a stuffed animal, are more common in people who are significantly destabilized and therefore require more rudimentary soothing activities. More typically, however, self-soothing involves doing things that produce positive and comforting sensory experiences; for example, taking a long, warm bath or shower; practicing yoga; going for a walk; eating (but not bingeing on) something especially enjoyable (e.g., a "comfort" food); playing a musical instrument; requesting a hug from a loved one; or getting a massage. Some people report that cuddling or petting a companion animal can be especially soothing. In some cases, those with childhood trauma may also gain from stimuli that convey positive attachment, for example, carrying around a smartphone recording of the client's therapist or close friend saying reassuring and affirming things that can be played as needed. In other cases, the client may be able to think of a person who has been kind and is loving, or who is a historic or spiritual figure associated with love, and imagine him or her, in detail, being present in the immediate moment, caring for the client.

Notably, some of self-soothing activities (e.g., taking a warm bath) cannot be engaged in immediately after one has been triggered. They are, however, potentially helpful in the hours after triggering has occurred, for example, when the person continues to struggle with activated thoughts, emotions, and memories into the night.

Strategic Distraction

Strategic distraction is, in a sense, similar to DRBs, except that the effect is rarely harmful, and it does not involve dramatic behaviors. Instead, the goal is to pull attention away from an activated internal state for a sufficient period of time, so that it fades for lack of reinforcement. Examples of strategic distraction following triggered distress include:

- Exercise
- Reading
- Conversations with safe/supportive others, including by cell phone when immediacy is important
- Listening to music
- Taking a "time-out" in a place or environment that feels more safe and is less triggering
- Interacting with, or cuddling, a pet
- Writing or journaling
- Going for a walk
- Engaging in yoga or *tai chi*.

It should be noted that distraction does not allow processing of triggered material, and may even have some suppression effects, although the latter are unknown. For this reason, although it can be effective in deescalating an immediately activated state, distraction should not be employed exclusive of other approaches and strategies.

Positive Self-Talk and Metacognitive Statements

Although often considered a sign of mental disturbance in popular culture, the cognitive literature indicates that we talk to ourselves on an ongoing basis (Azmitia, 1992). Researchers have especially identified *negative self-talk*, which involves internal monologues about one's failings, helplessness, guilt, shamefulness, unworthiness, or badness, as well as the dangerousness of the world and the hopelessness of the future. Such thoughts are especially common among those who were abused or neglected as children (Cloitre et al., 2006) and are associated with subsequent depression, anxiety, and posttraumatic stress (Kubany, Hill, & Owens, 2003; Lemoult, Kircanski, Prasad, & Gotlib, 2017; Yaratan & Yucesoylu, 2010). Most cognitive therapists suggest that negative self-talk is most detrimental when it is automatically assumed to be true and is therefore not internally disputed.

Positive self-talk, in contrast, is the antithesis of negative evaluations of self and the environment, because it focuses on the individual's positive qualities and intentions, self-efficacy, and entitlement to well-being and good treatment by others, as well as evaluation of the environment as safer than what negative self-talk portrays. In this sense, positive self-talk is not deliberate self-deception or empty affirmations, but rather, corrective responses to triggered beliefs that have been biased by abuse, neglect, insecure attachment, social marginalization, or more recent trauma.

Importantly, such activities require some degree of *metacognitive awareness* (Teasdale et al., 2002)—the realization that negative self-talk is just that, a monologue of devaluing and inaccurate evaluations that come from previous maltreatment or a harsh culture, as opposed to representing accurate perceptions of oneself, others, the environment, or the future. For this reason, teaching positive self-talk often involves discussion of the effects of early trauma and neglect on thinking, so that the client can appreciate why negative self-talk can be incorrect and should be argued against.

Early in treatment, DRB-involved clients can be encouraged to devise, then practice (initially out loud), positive self-statements that they can later call upon when triggered, such as the following:

- "I am a good person."
- "I'm doing the best I can."
- "As far as I can tell, I am safe."
- "I don't have to do this if I don't want to."
- "This is nothing to be ashamed of."
- "I can handle this."
- "I deserve respect."

He may also gain from practicing metacognitive statements such as the following:

- "This is just my past talking."
- "I'm just thinking _____ because of my childhood. It may not be true."
- "These are just thoughts, not facts."
- "These thoughts are from the past, but this isn't the past right now."
- "I don't have to believe what my mind is saying."

Initially, the client may have difficulty making these internal statements, either because they seem silly or child-like, or because she is not aware of her negative self-talk and therefore does not understand the need for a rebuttal. It is often best to acknowledge concerns about positive self-talk but suggest its value nevertheless. In many cases, the client slowly comes to appreciate the utility of this activity over time, as it is seen to decrease the power of triggered thoughts and feelings.

The following is an example of a more extended metacognitive self-discourse from a woman in therapy for depression who recently completed a mindfulness-based cognitive therapy course. As is apparent, she appears to have internalized and integrated a metacognitive perspective, to her benefit. She states:

> "It's hard to explain, but sometimes when I get the usual hit of how little I've done with my life, or about my weight, I just go 'yeah, yeah . . . talk, talk, talk.' I just let the thoughts go. Maybe you don't always have to fix what's happening in your mind, sometimes you can just let it do what it does, but say 'Hello, mind. You're in the past, poor mind, but this isn't the past right now.' . . . It's like, 'Hey mind, do whatever. But I don't have to believe what you're saying, at least not all the time.'" (in Briere, 2013, pp. 208–209)

Engaging in "Idealistic" (Najavits, 2002) or "Opposite-Action" (Linehan, 1993) Behaviors

In addition to positive self-talk, the client may find it helpful to respond to self-devaluation or demoralization with opposite behaviors that increase hope, perceived self-efficacy, and positive self-regard. For example, the client might consider:

- Doing people random favors, or helping strangers.
- Writing about his experiences, or doing other creative things that call on adversity to create something of meaning, value, or beauty.
- Practicing being kind to others, specifically at times when he feels resentment or anger.
- Doing something in the outside environment (e.g., volunteering) that increases feelings of competence or benevolence.

Focusing Mindful Attention on Triggered States

As described in detail in Chapter 7, and presented in Appendix 7, the client can use an exercise (ReGAIN) that increases mindfulness at the point of being triggered, and allows her, to some degree, to become more grounded, not resist triggered states, feel self-compassion, and lessen the need to reduce distress through a DRB.

Harm Reduction

Initially developed to address substance use, harm reduction is based on the notion that most of those who engage in unsafe behaviors are not intentionally trying to hurt themselves or others, but rather are unable or unwilling to stop a given behavior as a result of complex etiologies (including trauma), diverse motivations, and sometimes the effects of social deprivation and inequality. A harm reduction approach to self-endangering behaviors "work(s) to minimize [their] harmful effects rather than simply ignore or condemn them" (Harm Reduction Coalition, 2018, *http://harmreduction.org*, retrieved October 26, 2017). Notably, harm reduction does not ignore the real danger and debility associated with such behaviors (see *http://harmreduction.org/about-us/principles-of-harm-reduction*), but recognizes that reducing harm may be the best first option for those who cannot immediately discontinue self-endangering behavior.

In the context of the client who requires relatively extended treatment before she can discontinue self-endangering behavior, the issue is how to reduce the harmfulness of DRBs in the meantime. This is especially relevant to clients who have only recently entered treatment and who are experiencing acute levels of distress, instability, and, as a result, ongoing problematic behaviors.

Harm reduction approaches to DRBs generally involve:

• Attempting to delay avoidance behaviors for as long as possible after the onset of a trigger, so that (1) the associated distress goes unreinforced and potentially fades with time, and (2) the client has the opportunity to sit with, and develop greater emotional tolerance for, unwanted emotional states—both of which reduce the need for more powerful or harmful DRBs. This does not involve suppressing the urge to use a DRB in the future, but rather, allows the need to be present, but not immediately gratified.

• When some sort of behavior seems necessary, replacing dangerous DRBs with less detrimental ones, despite their less satisfactory nature—for example, doing push-ups beyond one's normal preference (but not harming oneself) or holding ice cubes until they hurt, instead of self-cutting. Notably, although such replacement activities are often recommended on self-help websites, they should only be used when absolutely necessary, and only in the context of immediate harm reduction—they are unlikely to resolve the underlying issues and, in some sense, they continue to model self-harm as a way to deal with self-injury.

• If the original DRB is impossible to avoid, consciously engaging in the behavior to the least extent possible (e.g., bingeing for 10 minutes rather than an hour, trying to limit sexual behavior to flirting as opposed to intercourse), so that the harmfulness of the behavior is reduced. These behaviors should be used judiciously, however, since (1) they may still be injurious or otherwise problematic, and (2) in some cases, lower-level involvement in a behavior (e.g., eating just one cookie) may trigger even more intense cravings or urges and thereby increase, not decrease, a DRB.

Together, relationship building, safety interventions, lessening trigger-related distress, and harm reduction activities offer the overwhelmed client the opportunity to understand and depathologize what have typically been experienced as shameful behaviors, increase his immediate safety, and begin to stabilize his internal environment. Because of the nature of DRBs and their underlying etiologies, however, these activities will have to be revisited at different times during treatment and should therefore be seen as cornerstones of effective therapy rather than just early stabilizing interventions.

CHAPTER 6

Acceptance and Mindfulness

Although current interventions for DRBs and other avoidance behaviors generally include some level of stabilization and attention to emotional regulation skills, many of them also teach nonresistance to painful internal states (e.g., Bowen, Chawla, & Marlatt, 2011; Habib et al., 2013; Hayes et al., 2012; Linehan, 1993). This is probably because distress avoidance tends to trigger the *suppression effect* (Briere, 2015): Although it is sometimes possible to suppress unwanted thoughts, feelings, and memories, such actions generally cause them to reappear later, sometimes with even greater frequency and intensity (Elliott & Briere, 1995; Taylor & Bryant, 2007; Roemer & Borkovec, 1994; Wegner, 1994). In other words, paradoxically, DRBs and other avoidance strategies may keep painful states alive into the long term, whereas their reverse—intentional acceptance of painful internal experience—may lead to decreased distress over time.

Mindfulness

Interestingly, although modern psychology has only recently discovered the negative effects of suppression, and the benefits of engaging distress, the Buddhist practice of *mindfulness* has endorsed this perspective for centuries. *Mindfulness,* which generally occurs in the context of meditation, may be defined as the ability to maintain ongoing awareness of—and openness to—one's moment-by-moment experience, including thoughts, emotions, perceptions, and memories, without judgment and with acceptance (for related definitions, see Germer, 2005, and Kabat-Zinn, 2003).

Central to this capacity is the ability to view one's internal experiences impartially, seeing them as neither good nor bad, and allowing them to come and go on their own—neither pushing them away nor being preoccupied with them. This process requires the ability to "let go": allowing thoughts and feelings into awareness, but not holding on to them or ruminating over them. Instead, mindfulness training teaches how to note a given experience, allow it to occur, but then attend to the next incoming thought, feeling, or memory, or—sometimes in meditation—return awareness to one's breath. Note that this is not a form of avoidance or suppression, but rather of freely shifting attention that, when done correctly, is not prone to suppression effects.

Given scientific findings on the unintended effects of avoidance, it is perhaps not surprising that mindfulness training has been found helpful in reducing many of the problems described in this book, including self-injury, eating disturbance, aggression, compulsive gambling, and suicidality, as well as correlates of these problems, including anxiety and depression, posttraumatic stress, dissociation, emotional dysregulation, and BPD (see meta-analyses on the clinical efficacy of mindfulness training; Coelho, Canter, & Ernst, 2007; Grossman, Neimann, Schmidt, & Walach, 2004; Hayes, Luoma, Bond, Masuda, & Lillis, 2006; Hofmann, Sawyer, Witt, & Oh, 2010; Khoury et al., 2013).

There are several possible explanations for why mindfulness might specifically decrease DRBs and other avoidance responses:

- Most directly, in the absence of avoidance, the suppression effect is not active; therefore, painful thoughts, feelings, and memories—although greater in the present moment—are less likely to reoccur later in time and thereupon motivate DRBs. As noted in this book, the choice to experience distress in the present, in the hope of less suffering in the future, can be a difficult one, especially for those struggling with acute attachment disturbance or trauma symptoms. Yet it is entirely possible with sufficient training and support.

- The increased acceptance and nonjudgment associated with mindfulness means that painful internal experiences are not seen as unacceptable or pathological. In a sense, distress experienced without the baggage of negative judgment is less "bad" and less likely to be less distressing, and therefore may require less avoidance.

- A mindful response to activated distress includes *metacognitive awareness:* the realization that feelings and thoughts are just that; psychological reactions to the environment and history that may or may not represent the true state of reality. Thus, for example, triggered anxiety can be seen as a subjectively unpleasant emotional state but not necessarily as evidence of current danger in the environment or the future. Similarly, a sudden intrusion of self-hatred would be understood as a painful cognitive–emotional experience, but not as information that one is actually bad, let alone hate-worthy. As a result, metacognitive awareness can lead to decreased reactivity—including a decreased tendency to respond with DRBs.

- Finally, triggered distress that is not resisted is, by definition, not avoided. Once allowed into awareness, the painful memories, thoughts, and feelings underlying DRBs are more available for psychological processing. As described in detail in Chapter 8, for example, anxiety associated with a traumatic memory can be lessened to the extent that it is evoked in relative safety, is not overwhelming, and is not avoided. Under such circumstances, extinction can occur—the memory of danger is activated, but is not reinforced, because the past has passed. And once triggering no longer produces distress, DRBs are less necessary.

Mindfulness Applications for DRBs

Taken together, the mindfulness literature reviewed earlier, and the experience of many empirically oriented clinicians (e.g., Habib et al., 2013; Orsillo & Batten, 2005; Semple & Madni, 2015; Follette, Briere, Rozelle, Hopper, & Rome, 2015; Wagner & Linehan, 2006) suggest the specific validity of mindfulness training in work with traumatized individuals. Fortunately, there are a number of validated mindfulness-related interventions that are relevant to survivors of attachment dysregulation and trauma, perhaps especially those involved in chronic DRBs. These include:

- DBT, which was specifically developed to assist those diagnosed with BPD who engage in DRBs (Linehan, 1993).
- ACT, which focuses on DRBs and other experiential avoidance behaviors.
- Mindfulness-based relapse prevention (MBRP; Bowen et al., 2011), which targets problematic substance use.
- Two popular and well-validated mindfulness-based training packages, both of which has been specifically adapted for trauma survivors (Dutton, 2015; Kimbrough, Magyari, Langenberg, Chesney, & Berman, 2010; Magyari, 2015; Semple & Madni, 2015):
  - Mindfulness-based stress reduction (MBSR; Kabat-Zinn, 1982)
  - Mindfulness-based cognitive therapy (MBCT; Segal, Williams, & Teasdale, 2002)

Yet, although DBT and ACT successfully integrate elements of mindfulness into their treatment models, and MBRP, MBSR, and MBCT are clearly relevant to trauma survivors, there are several issues associated with combining mindfulness training into DRB-focused psychotherapy, including the following:

- The likelihood that significant amounts of mindfulness training (e.g., at the level provided by MBSR, MBCT, or MBRP groups) are required to produce the magnitude of effects on DRBs reported in the mindfulness outcome literature.
- The complexities associated with adapting group-oriented, non-clinically focused mindfulness training procedures to individual, process-oriented, relational psychotherapy for attachment- and trauma-related difficulties.
- The probability that most psychotherapists have insufficient training or experience in mindfulness interventions to support their teaching mindfulness to clients in treatment.
- The reality that the most immediately important aspects of therapy for many trauma survivors is not mindfulness per se, but rather safety, stabilization, developing a strong therapeutic relationship, and building emotional regulation capacities. In this context, the time and energy required to teach the client mindfulness skills, at least beyond simple breathing exercises, might easily interfere with, or supplant, these more central treatment components—at least in the early phases of therapy.

A Hybrid Approach

These various issues seem to present a conundrum: Mindfulness is obviously relevant to a variety of problems experienced by DRB-involved clients, yet (1) many clinicians are not fully prepared to teach mindfulness to their clients, and (2) despite the helpfulness of mindfulness skills, learning them may be problematic when doing so interferes with more immediately important therapeutic tasks.

Given these issues, mindfulness training may be best employed as an add-on to ongoing treatment, in which the client is referred to an established mindfulness training center while, at the same time, receiving separate psychotherapy. For example, if economics and geography allow, a client undergoing DRB-oriented treatment also might be referred to a center providing MBSR, MBRP, or MBCT.

This hybrid approach, described in more detail elsewhere (e.g., Briere, 2015; Briere & Scott, 2014) involves the following steps:

- *Screen for the appropriateness of mindfulness training.* As noted, DRB-involved clients are often subject to easily triggered attachment- and trauma-related memories, often in the context of reduced emotional regulation capacities. Because meditation and mindfulness reduce avoidance, and encourage inwardly focused attention, they can lead to greater exposure to painful memories and emotional states (Germer, 2005; Hayes et al., 2012; Treanor, 2011). In most cases, this increased exposure is not overwhelming or harmful—hence the wide participation of trauma survivors in North American mindfulness trainings and retreats (Kornfield, 1993), and the effectiveness of DBT, ACT, and other mindfulness-oriented interventions for trauma survivors (Follette et al., 2015).

Nevertheless, because DRBs often signal emotional instability, it is important that screening be done before mindfulness training is considered. Most obviously, clients experiencing psychosis, severe depression, mania, or significant suicidality should typically avoid meditation-based mindfulness training until these symptoms or conditions are resolved or under better control. The reader is referred to Germer (2005) for suggestions regarding screening and the use of mindfulness with symptomatic trauma survivors.

• *If indicated, consider alternatives to mindfulness training.* When screening indicates that mindfulness is not immediately appropriate, other, less internally focused contemplative activities may still prove helpful. Less activating approaches often include trauma-sensitive yoga (Emerson, 2015), lovingkindness meditations (Salzberg, 2002), and self-compassion exercises (Germer & Neff, 2015). Notably, however, trauma survivors who are especially consumed by low self-esteem or shame sometimes may respond with fear, anger, or avoidance to suggestions that they be more kind or compassionate toward themselves (Germer & Neff, 2015; Gilbert, 2010). Such reactions highlight the need to tailor interventions— even those thought to be benign—to the specific difficulties and concerns of each client.

• *If the client can tolerate it, and the therapist has had some training in meditation, teach elementary meditation techniques,* for example, the breath counting exercise presented in Appendix 1. This can be done with only minimal (but necessary) therapist expertise and, especially for those who do not want to engage in more formal mindfulness activities, can be helpful during RA-focused treatment. If use of the *meditation* label is problematic for the client (i.e., the client thinks it is too "New Age," culturally or religiously incompatible, or frightening for some reason), just refer to the Appendix 1 exercise as deep relaxation or mindful breath training.

• *Refer those clients who wish to learn more extended mindfulness to an MBSR, MBCT, or MBRP group.* Generally, these classes involve six to eight weekly sessions of 1–2 hours' duration, daily meditation sessions at home, homework assignments, and a daylong retreat. In these groups, attendees specifically learn to practice mindfulness meditation, including:

○ Focusing their attention on a single target (e.g., the breath or sensations in the body), and when the mind is distracted by thoughts, emotions, or sensations, noting these intrusions in a nonjudgmental way, then returning to the target of attention.

o *Body scans,* in which participants are led through a guided, progressive exploration of bodily sensations.

o Gentle stretching and Hatha yoga positions.

o Teaching and group discussions on mindfulness, meditation, and mind-related contributions to stress.

o In addition, MBCT especially focuses on developing metacognitive awareness, and MBRP adds, among other things, training on *urge surfing,* described below.

• *As the client gains meditation and mindfulness skills–ideally through outside training, but also through exercises like those presented in Appendix 1– these capacities can be called upon during DRB-focused psychotherapy, to the extent that the clinician him- or herself is mindfulness-informed.* This includes the following:

o *Settling skills.* Meditation can teach the client to down-regulate her anxiety or hyperarousal (Baer, 2003; Ogden, Minton, & Pain, 2000), which can then be applied in treatment and the outside world at times of triggered distress.

o *The ability to "let go" of persistent internal phenomena.* The capacity to redirect, but not suppress, awareness and attention can be helpful when the client encounters upsetting thoughts, feelings, or memories in treatment—and in life—that otherwise might lead to preoccupation, obsession, or rumination.

o *Accessing the exposure component of mindfulness.* The decreased avoidance associated with mindfulness may allow the emergence of previously suppressed or inhibited trauma or attachment memories and their emotional sequelae (Briere, 2015). In the context of a relatively relaxed state and a less involved, nonjudgmental, and accepting cognitive perspective (Baer, 2003; Germer, 2005), this process can allow desensitization of attachment- or trauma-related memories.

o *Metacognitive awareness.* During mindfulness training, the client learns to consider his trauma-related negative cognitions, feelings, and memories as "just" products of the mind (i.e., reexperienced history that is not necessarily real in the current context). In therapy (and outside of it), this new perspective may allow the client to change her relationship to triggered thoughts and feelings, such that they are no longer experienced as harbingers of actual danger or self-inadequacy.

o *Urge surfing.* An integral part of MBRP, the client may learn to apply mindfulness skills to sudden, often trauma- or attachment-related, urges to engage in a DRB or other avoidance behavior. Reflecting

Kabat-Zinn's (1994) reminder that "you can't stop the waves, but you can learn to surf" (p. 32), the survivor is encouraged to see the need to engage in a DRB as similar to riding a wave: The need starts small, builds in size, peaks, then, if not avoided or held onto, slowly falls away. If the client can view these needs as temporary intrusions that can be ridden like a surfboard—neither fought against nor acted upon—she may be able to avoid using a DRB despite being triggered.

Mindfulness and DRBs Revisited

Because mindfulness is, to some extent, the antithesis of avoidance, it can be a valuable addition to DRB-focused therapy. However, not all clients want to learn mindfulness skills. In fact, some may see mindfulness—like other awareness-building tools—as a direct threat to the best defenses against distress that they possess. Others may have religious or cultural objections to mindfulness training, even when it is framed from a non-sectarian perspective. As well, some clients do not have geographic or financial access to mindfulness training, although mindfulness centers are proliferating and increasingly provide services to those with limited or no funds.

For these reasons, the hybrid mindfulness approach to therapy is not always possible. When this is true, the clinician who regularly sees DRB-involved clients might consider taking a mindfulness class, ideally followed by additional training, so that some aspects of mindfulness can be a part of their treatment repertoire. Minimally, to the extent that the clinician can teach the client simple meditation and mindfulness skills—however they are introduced or labeled—the client may learn to ground and settle himself when encountering triggers or triggered states, and develop metacognitive skills that decrease reactivity.

Equally important, beyond teaching the client mindfulness skills, the mindfulness-trained therapist herself may become more self-aware, accepting, and compassionate (Germer & Siegel, 2014). From that position, she may be better able to respond to challenging client behaviors without reactivity or counteractivation, instead offering the compassion, attunement, and positive regard often associated with positive treatment outcomes (Germer & Siegel, 2014; Rogers, 1957).

CHAPTER 7

Trigger Management

Because triggers play a critical role in the development of DRBs, RA-focused treatment emphasizes the importance of identifying, intervening in, and reducing their effects. *Trigger management* occurs when the client:

- Becomes aware of triggers, their etiology, and their role in DRBs
- Is able to identify when triggering has occurred
- Discovers what internal and external stimuli lead to triggering
- Works to reduce the effects of triggering, so that DRBs become unnecessary or are less frequent or extreme.

Several trigger-related approaches were described in Chapter 5, primarily as they support increased safety and emotional stability during the early stages of treatment. In this chapter, trigger management is outlined more formally, especially as it is used once stabilization has occurred.

Psychoeducation on Triggers and Triggering

Clinical experience suggests that many clients who are triggered into DRBs are not aware of having been triggered. There are a number of possible reasons for this, including the likelihood that, as noted earlier, some avoidance responses are so effective that they block awareness of their existence, let alone their etiology. As well, there are significant cultural differences in how traumatic events are understood (Marsella, Friedman, Gerrity, & Scurfield, 1996). For example, not all people in North America or Europe are conversant with, or endorse, therapist-driven ideas involving trauma or triggering. And as many working in refugee or immigrant mental health centers will attest, a number of world cultures do not have models of distress that include such ideas, or, if they do, they are represented in divergent frames of reference (Briere & Scott, 2014).

Even more relevant may be the effects of *source attribution errors* (Briere & Scott, 2014) in the triggering process. Often applied in memory research, this term refers to situations in which people believe their experiences come from one source, but, in fact, they come from somewhere else. In the trauma context, implicit memories are typically not experienced as memories when they are triggered, but rather are "relived" as perceptions of the immediate environment. As a result, the triggered individual may attribute his sudden rage or feelings of abandonment to the people around him rather than to triggered memories of past maltreatment or attachment disturbance. For example, a minor disagreement with a friend might trigger strong, abuse-related feelings of criticism or rejection, and the person may interpret these feelings as due to the friend's behavior rather than to activated implicit memories of childhood. In this event, the person might deny that she was triggered but note that she has some mean friends.

What Is Real and What Is Not

Psychoeducation about the effects of avoidance on awareness, and the existence of source attribution errors, can be a helpful early step on the path to trigger management. At the same time, this information is potentially unsettling, since it implies that what one thinks one knows may not be true. The client may believe that she is not avoiding, largely because she is doing such a good job of it. And as a result of source attribution errors, her perceptions of internal cause and effect may not be accurate. To further complicate matters, seeing things as they actually are can, at least initially, invite further distress: Reduced avoidance means allowing pain that has been held at bay, and correcting source attribution errors means confronting past trauma and its persistence over time. Finally, an understanding of trigger dynamics can lead to a paradoxical realization: Doing things to feel better may actually make things worse, whereas letting oneself feel unwanted things may reduce distress in the long term (Briere & Scott, 2014).

Despite these challenges, the benefits of psychoeducation are clear. As the client comes to recognize triggers in the environment, knows what to expect when triggering occurs, and learns ways of responding to triggered states, the world may become less chaotic and more predictable, and her sense of self-efficacy may increase.

These insights and understandings often emerge naturally as a function of RA-focused treatment and psychoeducation, but they also may be increased as the client completes the *Functions of Distress Reduction Behaviors* (F-DRB) worksheet (see Appendix 4), wherein the specific reasons for the client's DRBs are explored. For example, if the client reports on the F-DRB that he engages in self-injury as a way to distract himself from triggered memories of sexual abuse, the internal logic of self-harm can become more apparent, and potentially less associated with shame or pathology.

Given these issues, it is helpful to explore trigger dynamics and functions with DRB-involved clients. Generally, this discussion includes the following points:

- Childhood memories of abuse or attachment disturbance often last into the long term.
- Early childhood memories (i.e., in the first 3 or 4 years) often cannot be voluntarily recalled, but they can be triggered by reminiscent stimuli in the current environment, at which point they appear as sudden, real-time, emotions, sensations, and thoughts.
- Triggered thoughts or feelings tend to be attributed to whatever triggered them, such as an argument or an experience of rejection.
- If the memory or the feelings are overwhelming, people sometimes engage in behaviors such as indiscriminate sexual activities, aggression, or self-injury as a way to avoid or reduce emotional distress.
- Unfortunately, these behaviors not only can be dangerous or life-threatening, they rarely work in the long-term. Instead, suppressed or avoided distress tends to return as intrusive thoughts and emotions, flashbacks, sudden feelings of shame, or unwanted memories, often leading to more DRBs.

As noted elsewhere, psychoeducation is often least effective when it involves lecturing the client or merely providing written materials (Becker, Rankin, & Rickel, 1998; Briere, 2004). Instead, understanding may best emerge in the context of a two-way conversation in which the client explores trigger dynamics with the therapist, and calls on her own experiences with triggering and its relationship to DRBs. Although it might be assumed that the average client would be unable to understand implicit memories, triggers, or DRBs, this is not necessarily the case. Much of the RA perspective makes sense to traumatized people who have been triggered in the past, especially when the clinician avoids jargon, conveys respect for the client's personal experiences, presents it in a culturally relevant way, and makes sure that the material is understood and can be integrated into the client's actual life. In some cases, it may take additional time for these ideas to be conveyed, especially if trauma, major source attribution errors, cultural differences, cognitive impairment, or the effects of social marginalization (e.g., distrust, educational deprivation) are present.

Direct and Indirect Trigger Identification

Following some level of psychoeducation, trigger identification occurs when the client is able to identify times when he has been triggered, and to relate triggered states to specific triggers. Triggers can be identified in two ways:

1. Because they are obvious and can be verbally described (e.g., sexual stimuli triggering memories of child sexual abuse).
2. Because the client becomes aware of an atypical state (e.g., sudden dissociation, dizziness, or intrusive self-denigrating thoughts) after encountering a newly present stimulus (e.g., being yelled at, feeling rejected), and thereby discovers a new trigger.

Direct Identification

When a trigger is already known to the client, and it is present at the same time as an urge to engage in a DRB, it may be relatively easy for him to determine that triggering has occurred, and respond accordingly. For this reason, trigger management usually begins with the client identifying as many triggers as possible on the Trigger Review (TR; see Appendix 3), for example, angry faces, criticism, sexual stimuli, yelling, perceived rejection or abandonment, authority figures, the smell of alcohol, or boundary violations. Often, the TR worksheet expands over time: At the onset of treatment, the client may only be able to identify one or two triggers but may discover more as therapy progresses and she encounters other stimuli that reveal themselves to be triggers. For example, a sexual abuse survivor might initially identify sexual activities and stimuli as triggers for anger, revulsion, and shame, but later discover that she is also triggered by being disbelieved or not taken seriously, boundary violations, and perceived abandonment by parental figures.

As the client is increasingly able to identify when she is being triggered, she has more opportunities to develop metacognitive awareness, as described in Chapter 6. For example, someone with a history of witnessing domestic violence as a child may learn that interpersonal conflict triggers feelings of helplessness and anger. As a result, although triggered by an argument, the client may become aware that he is not "really" mad about what is currently happening, but rather is being triggered by it.

And if, in fact, there is little to be upset about in the current context (e.g., "just" an argument vs. physical violence), immediate anger or fear may lessen, reducing the likelihood or intensity of a DRB.

Habitual DRBs, Trigger Generalization, and Trigger Chains

In some cases, when avoidance behaviors are chronic, the connection between previously directly identified triggers and current DRBs may become harder to track over time. For example, a client may initially self-injure because of intrusive memories of sexual and emotional abuse, but eventually respond to any current distress or dysphoria, irrespective of its genesis, with self-injury or another DRB.

When the client has great difficulty tracing current distress to a specific triggered memory, or there are many potential triggers for the same response, the therapist may consider treating antecedent negative thoughts or feelings, whatever their source, as triggers, since they have become disconnected from their original trauma or attachment etiology. Thus, for example, the client might learn to identify emotional or cognitive precursors (e.g., shame or helplessness) to compulsive sexual behavior, and practice metacognitive responses to these phenomena, with less reference to the sexual abuse that initially motivated these unwanted intrusions. At the same time, however, it is recommended that trigger identification activities continue to be revisited on occasion, in case (or until) the client can become more aware of the actual etiology of her DRBs.

Indirect Identification

Indirect identification occurs when the client infers that she has been triggered, based on her reactions in the moment. This process is often necessary when the client is not yet aware of a specific trigger, or even that he has been triggered in the first place. For example, a person might engage in a dramatic behavior but erroneously attribute it to something in the environment rather than to a triggered memory, and thus miss the chance to problem-solve and reduce his reactivity.

Indirect identification involves two steps:

1. Recognition that one is in a suddenly changed state (e.g., involving disproportionate anger, panic, sudden hypervigilance, or dissociation).
2. Investigation of what has activated that state (e.g., an interaction with someone who reminds the client of a previous abuser or traumatic event).

Discovery that something has changed is facilitated by mindfulness of one's immediate internal experiences and growing awareness of how triggering generally feels. In some cases, triggered states are accompanied by dissociation and/or disorganized thinking, so that it is difficult for the client to know exactly what she is experiencing. Mindfulness training can help the client attend to internal experience more easily, even during times of emotional activation, and therefore be better able to notice that he is in a different cognitive–emotional state than minutes before.

When the client is able to recognize that something has changed internally, the next step is usually to determine whether these changes, in fact, signal triggering. Based on experience with a precursor to the measure developed for this book (The Trigger Grid; Briere & Lanktree, 2012), there appear to be a number of specific reactions that individuals commonly have when they have been triggered. These include the following:

- Contextually inappropriate or overintense emotions or behaviors (e.g., being more angry, frightened, or sad than would make sense for the situation, or suddenly feeling self-hatred or shame for no obvious reason).
- Intrusive thoughts that seem to be more relevant to the past— whether based on trauma or harsh social messages—than the present (e.g., "He's making a fool of me"; "I have to get even"; "This is my fault"; or "I am such a _____").
- Brief dissociative responses (e.g., "spacing out," out-of-body experiences, numbing, altered perceptions).
- Feeling younger, as if one were a child.
- Having *déjà vu* experiences (e.g., "This has happened before").
- Microflashbacks (e.g., very rapid, often fragmentary images, sounds, or sensations associated with past traumas).
- Somatic reactions (e.g., sudden flushing, tightened scalp, dizziness, shortness of breath, rapid respirations, or tachycardia).

These and other trigger-suggestive responses can be queried by the therapist or spontaneously volunteered by the client, or they can be prompted by use of the Trigger Review. Although this tool asks about cognitive, emotional, or somatic reactions associated with already identified triggers, the resultant list of trigger-related phenomena can be used by the client to identify triggered states in the future.

Once indirect identification indicates that the client is (or was) in a triggered state, the goal is to identify the specific trigger(s) involved, either at the time of the triggering or later in the therapy session. This may occur through detailed discussions with the clinician about the events that led up to the altered state, often guided by the TR. For example, the client might identify a situation (e.g., a loud party), a specific stimulus (e.g., a leering face), or a personal interaction (e.g., being "hit on") that transpired just before she became dissociated, fearful, or aggressive.

Pausing the Process

It is important to recognize that some clients are not able to move immediately from identification to the next step in trigger management process—trigger linkage—because they are overwhelmed by activated distress. When this occurs, the client should be reminded that being able to detect triggering is a tremendous step forward. Because of source attribution errors and trigger chaining, many people who are triggered never discover that they are responding to distant memories, not actual current events, and, thus, have a harder time controlling what happens afterward. When the client has reached this milestone, her primary task is now to problem-solve ways to reduce the effects of triggers and thereby forestall DRBs. It may only be later, once emotional regulation capacities have been improved, that the next step in the process can occur.

Trigger–Trauma Linkage

When the client is ready and able, linking a trigger to memory of a specific event or events can further metacognitive awareness. For example, connecting a trigger to a prior trauma might support the metacognitive self-statement "This isn't about [the current circumstance], it is about [a particular past event]," the specificity of which may make it easier for the client to see that, in fact, his current emotions or thoughts arise from a memory, not from a current event.

The process of connecting triggers to memories is referred to as *trigger–trauma linkage* in RA-focused treatment. This can be facilitated through use of the Triggers-to-Memories Worksheet (TMW; see Appendix 5), which asks the client to connect specific triggers directly to specific memories, generally of childhood maltreatment or attachment disturbance, although sometimes adult traumas. For example, the client might link being triggered by people yelling to psychological and physical abuse by a parent, or identify sexual triggers that connect to memories of sexual victimization.

In other cases, however, the triggered memories may be implicit, in which case they cannot be verbally identified. For example, the client might be triggered by a loved one's seemingly dismissive behavior, and not be able to link it with a specific memory of early neglect by an attachment figure. Yet, as noted earlier, even in the case of triggered implicit memories, the client and therapist may be able to hypothesize [but not prove] early abuse or neglect based on later autobiographical memories (e.g., projecting backwards based on explicit memories of uninvolved caretaking or physical abuse at age 4 or 5); thus, trigger–trauma linkage may still be approximated.

Finally, when trigger chaining is a major issue, use of the TMW may become more complicated. In some cases, as described in Chapter 5, the client may report that difference instances of the same trigger lead to a variety of different memories, thoughts, and feelings. In such instances, the clinician might suggest that the client indicate as many traumas as he can recall for each trigger listed on the TMW. Thus, the individual might indicate that perceived criticism is a major trigger, then indicate a variety of trauma memories that arise when she is triggered by judgments from others, for example, instances of parental psychological abuse, being blamed for having been sexually abused as a child, and harsh statements from an abusive boyfriend or girlfriend in adolescence.

Whether the memories associated with a given trigger are implicit or explicit, autobiographically accessed or reexperienced, linked or otherwise, the process of connecting triggers to memories can help the client develop a coherent, nonpathologizing narrative regarding his early experiences and current DRBs. It also reinforces the metacognitive notion that memories can masquerade as real experiences, and the past can seem like the present.

Intervening in Triggered States in Order to Reduce DRBs

As the client develops greater awareness of her particular triggers, the negative experiences that fuel them, and the painful states they produce, her relationship to triggered experiences often changes. The transition from "perceiving" to "remembering" carries with it the growing realization that thoughts and feelings do not always represent accurate information about the here and now. Most importantly, if one's perceptions are actually intrusions of the past, there may, in fact, be nothing to be upset about in the present moment.

At the same time, trigger awareness may be only part of what the client needs to counter DRBs. In the following example, Sacha, who has been in over a year of RA-focused trauma therapy, is involved in the following trigger and response:

- "I am really pissed off. He talked to me like I was a [expletive] kid, said my work was [expletive]."
- "But I gotta chill. This is the kind of situation where I lose it. And this is intense. Am I getting triggered again?"
- "These feelings are way out of control. Big deal, he just said my project needs work. So what? But I'm pissed off. My heart is racing, I'm tense, the way I get."

- "One of my biggest triggers is here: Put down by an old guy, like he knows what the [expletive] he's talking about. He and my dad would be great pals."
- "I'm definitely triggered."
- "I can't help it. I need to mess this guy up. He deserves it, and it'll feel good. But this is a triggered thing. It's just thoughts, not facts. And I'll lose this job."
- "OK, this isn't real. There's not really anything going on. He's my boss, he gets to give me feedback. This is dad stuff. But my dad isn't here, and this guy doesn't have a knife. I need to chill."

Although Sacha has done well in terms of identifying triggers, linking his emotional and cognitive responses to memories of his abusive father, and giving himself metacognitive advice, will this be enough?

The answer may be "yes" for those whose metacognitive awareness is sufficient to deescalate triggered states. But, in other cases, more may be required. As described in Chapter 5, trigger management also involves learning specific skills to "bring down" triggered states once they have occurred. They include:

- *Actions that immediately address triggered responses,* such as grounding, mindful breathing and muscle relaxation, self-soothing, and strategic distraction.
- *Positive self-talk and metacognitive statements* that counter negative self-appraisals and source attribution errors, and tend to self-validate and soothe.
- *Counterbehaviors,* including idealistic and opposite actions, that activate intentions and hopes that are contrary to activated states and potential DRBs.
- *Pre- and posttrigger activities* that decrease reactivity in general, such as meditation and mindfulness training.

In the previous example, Sacha might follow his trigger awareness with behaviors he learned in therapy:

- "OK, take a deep breath, let it go. Gotta breathe, in and out. One more time, follow the breath, in and out . . ."
- "This is just my past talking, everything's fine right now . . . Check out the room, notice the walls, the furniture . . . In and out . . . Don't have to do anything, anger is just a feeling . . . Let it come, let it go . . . Maybe count to 10 . . ."
- "I'm better at this stuff than I used to be . . . I don't have to do anything right now, just let it go. He's just a jerk. I can handle this. I got this . . . In and out, follow the breath. Let it go, relax. Look around the room."

- "Maybe turn this around. Thank him for the feedback. I don't have to be the hard guy."
- "Naw, he's an [expletive]."
- "OK, maybe a compromise. How could I improve this project? Show him what good work looks like. Or whatever. Be better than him. Which isn't that hard . . . All right, he's not that bad. He's just being a boss, it's his job. I'd like to be a boss someday, too."

Sacha's responses highlight the central aspects of trigger management:

- Recognize that triggering has occurred.
- Do what is necessary not to be overwhelmed by triggered responses, generally by grounding oneself.
- To the extent possible, accept the associated thoughts and feelings without acting on them.
- Identify the triggers and their links to memories.
- Develop metacognitive awareness of the difference between triggered memories and accurate perceptions of the present.

RAINing and ReGAINing

Interestingly, Buddhist mindfulness teachers have long discussed aspects of trigger management, although they generally speak of addressing reactivity. In fact, as described below, there is a mindfulness approach that closely parallels several of the interventions described in this book. Referred to as *RAIN*, this well-known technique was first developed by meditation teacher Michele McDonald (*https://learn.tricycle.org/courses/rain*), and later expanded and popularized by Buddhist psychologist Tara Brach (2013).[1] The acronym refers to four suggested steps in responding to an upsetting experience: **Re**cognize, **A**llow, **I**nvestigate, and **N**onidentify.

The RAIN algorithm is widely taught in mindfulness classes as a way for people to decrease their reactivity to internal or external events. It is slightly adapted here for use with those who are prone to triggering, and who, in the absence of sufficient emotional regulation skills, tend to respond with DRBs. This modified RAIN approach is renamed *ReGAIN*, because it adds a grounding step between *Recognize* and *Allow*. It also emphasizes, much as Brach (2013) does for RAIN, the need for the client to do only what is possible in the moment, without being overwhelmed.

---

[1]Tara Brach's many podcasts are highly recommended for both therapists and clients. They can be located at *www.tarabrach.com/talks-audio-video*.

ReGAIN may be relatively easy to remember, in that it suggests regaining one's balance, equanimity, or functioning after being triggered into a challenging state.

ReGAIN consists of the following steps, although it is common for someone to follow any given step with an earlier one, then perhaps skip to a later one; the process is not always linear:

- *Re*cognize that you are triggered.
- *G*round yourself.
- As best you can, *A*llow yourself to experience whatever is coming up, with self-compassion.
- *I*nvestigate how you are triggered, where the thoughts or feelings come from, and why they make you upset.
- *N*onidentify: Remind yourself that these experiences aren't real; they are just triggered thoughts, feelings, or memories. They aren't you; they are just what you are experiencing.

Because this is a tool that the client can carry with her, it is provided in Appendix 7 and is available online to purchasers of this book (see the box at the end of the table of contents).

Before ReGAINing is discussed in detail, its paradoxical nature should be acknowledged. Although this technique is ultimately associated with less suffering over time, its primary action derives from nonavoidance, and exploration of challenging experiences. As a result, some clients who are early in the treatment process may experience an increase in distress when first practicing the *recognizing* and/or *allowing* components of this exercise. This can be mitigated by inviting the client to initially practice ReGAIN on a more superficial level—acknowledging emergent unwanted states, but not fully engaging them—until she has gained the emotional regulation capacity required for more "deep" versions of this exercise.

The original RAIN approach invites the individual to be aware of, open to, and interested in all ongoing experiences, albeit especially difficult ones. The ReGAIN version presented here is specific to triggered states, and proceeds as follows:

- *Re*cognize **that something has happened and that you are probably in a triggered state.** Originally presented as *Recognize what is happening* (Brach, 2013), this step refers to being aware that something has changed internally, that one is having emotions, thoughts, sensations, or memories that were not present moments before. Unfortunately, people who engage in dissociation, thought suppression, denial, or excessive substance use may be relatively unaware of their ongoing experience, including whether it has changed. In the absence of such information, the client may not notice that he has been triggered, and will have fewer opportunities to intervene in impending DRBs.

Recognition therefore relies on some degree of mindfulness: the ability to be aware of moment-by-moment experiences without interference—to be able to know, and name, what is happening internally without self-judgment. As noted, this capacity also benefits from reduced substance use or dissociation, to the extent that the client has control over those phenomena. Of course, such awareness also can have a downside, since it involves increased access to unwanted thoughts, feelings, and memories. This means that the client who is beleaguered by upsetting internal events, often in the presence of reduced emotional regulation skills, may need to approach the *Recognition* phase of ReGAIN with care and self-compassion.

Beyond increasing mindfulness, those who have difficulty recognizing changed states can use a self-observation approach, referred to as *emotional detective work* (Briere & Lanktree, 2012). In this activity, the client learns to notice bodily cues signaling emotional arousal or distress, such as increased heart rate, shortness of breath, flushing, coldness of extremities, scalp tightness, restlessness, or clenched muscles, along with emergent thoughts and microflashbacks, to infer the intrusion of emotions or memories. Since, for many, awareness of the body is more grounding and less distressing than awareness of thoughts or feelings, this approach may serve as a "work-around" for some clients, until more emotional regulation and mindfulness is available.

Again, Recognition can be challenging, especially for those who don't, in fact, want to recognize that they are upset. As a result, the client must be patient with herself as she slowly grows this capacity. Equally important, the therapist should be sure to praise and validate the client for the bravery entailed in paying attention when not doing so may be more comfortable and less challenging.

• **_Ground_ yourself.** This step, not included in the traditional RAIN procedure, encourages the client to engage in activities that allow greater stability and self-support when experiencing the immediate effects of having been triggered. It is added in ReGAIN because, as noted throughout this book, it is not unusual for survivors of trauma or adverse attachment experiences to be overwhelmed by triggered states, and thus require some stabilization before actually addressing activated feelings, emotions, and memories.

Similar to "pausing the process" in trigger management, *grounding* includes activities such as slowing one's breath, practicing mindfulness or a brief breath/relaxation exercise, engaging in metacognitive self-talk, using strategic distraction, and attending to the here and now (vs. the there and then of triggered states).

Once the client is sufficiently grounded and deescalated, he can move onto the next step, *Allowing.*

• ***As best you can, Allow yourself to experience whatever is coming up, with self-compassion.*** Brach (2013) refers to this step as *Allowing life to be just as it is.* In RA-focused therapy, the goal is slightly more circumscribed, in that it calls for specific acceptance of triggered experiences. In this context, "allowing" refers to nonresistance—to the extent possible, not fighting, suppressing, or otherwise avoiding suddenly arising internal states, but instead allowing them to occur.

Because allowing such experiences can be difficult, this step also includes *self-compassion:* appreciation of how difficult it can be to sit with triggered emotions, thoughts, and memories, and the bravery associated with allowing these experiences to occur without pushing them away. As Kristin Neff (*http://self-compassion.org/the-three-elements-of-self-compassion-2*) notes, "Instead of just ignoring your pain with a 'stiff upper lip' mentality, you stop to tell yourself 'this is really difficult right now,' how can I comfort and care for myself in this moment?" Self-compassion may involve the affirming self-statements described in Chapter 5, but more generally it invites the person to feel caring and appreciation for herself in the same way she would feel compassion for someone else who was "in her shoes" and going through the same thing. Importantly, self-compassion is not used in this step to alter or reduce newly allowed thoughts or feelings, but rather to provide a stabilizing base of self-acceptance and appreciation when triggered states arise in the mind or body.

Since those involved in habitual DRBs, by definition, use avoidance as a primary survival strategy, allowing unwanted memories and associated feelings can be challenging. For this reason, RA clients are encouraged not only to practice self-compassion but also to experiment with titrating awareness: not only "letting in" thoughts or feelings, at whatever level is tolerable but also having the option to stop doing so if the experience become overwhelming. As well, the client may gain from returning to the ReGAIN *Grounding* step—for example, using self-soothing and breathing techniques to help her remain "present" during this step.

The benefits of *allowing* are several:

○ The suppression effect, which occurs when internal phenomena are avoided or blocked, is no longer as active; thus, emotional distress is less likely to endure into the long-term.

○ Learning to "sit with" unwanted experiences even briefly teaches nonresistance and distress tolerance (Linehan, 1993), and builds emotional regulation capacity, which reduces the need for avoidance responses such as DRBs and excessive substance use.

○ Memories and emotions that are allowed to emerge unimpeded, and are associated with self-compassion, can be processed and counter-conditioned over time. As trauma or attachment memories lose their ability to produce extreme distress, the client has less need for avoidance, including DRBs.

○ Practicing self-compassion at times of triggered distress allows the client to more deeply learn self-acceptance, since it is evoked on a regular basis and often proves helpful in the context of invalidating, self-hating, or shaming thoughts and feelings.

• _Investigate_ **how you have been triggered, the source of the trigger, and the source of the suffering.** This step, which is an adaptation of what Brach (2013) calls _Investigate inner experience with kindness,_ varies to some extent from the original Buddhist meaning. In Buddhist psychology, _investigation_ usually means the process of uncovering what one is preoccupied with, or "attached" to, so that one can let go of these desires and suffer less from unmet needs. Although this meaning is not overlooked from an RA perspective, the ReGAIN version of RAIN is more directly concerned with the triggering process. Among the questions that can be investigated are those discussed in this chapter, including:

○ "What is triggering me?"

○ "Why is it happening right now"

○ "Where do these triggers come from?"

• At the same time, inquiry may include another, more existential question:

○ "Why does this triggered experience hurt so much?"

• Among the answers that investigation might point to include:

○ _The effects of trauma and attachment disturbance:_ "I was really hurt by what happened (or in the case of attachment issues, often by what didn't happen), perhaps more than I realized, and the pain is still alive and well, even though I wish that it wasn't."

○ _The effects of harsh social messages:_ "These memories come with beliefs that I am bad, unlovable, and unworthy, which sometimes hurt as much or more than what happened to me."

○ _The effects of culturally supported unrealistic expectations:_ "I have been trained to want to be perfect, intelligent, likable, successful, and conventionally attractive, so when memories of trauma or abuse suggest I'm not those things, I suffer even more."

○ _The effects of resistance:_ "Trying to not feel or think about the past doesn't work; it makes it worse, unpredictable, and more likely to come back."

- As Brach (2013) notes more generally, it is important that the client know that the *Investigation* step does not involve evaluation of her weaknesses, problems, or symptoms, but rather is a self-compassionate examination of triggers and their effects. The underlying message remains that triggering is due to previous negative experiences beyond the client's control; it does not signal personal failings or psychological disorder.

In fact, investigation may to some extent be a prerequisite for self-compassion: the client can rarely "just" access self-acceptance or self-forgiveness solely because it someone has suggested that she do so. Rather, self-acceptance generally arises from insight, especially the realization that one is not inherently unacceptable or unworthy, but, instead, has been attempting to survive the effects of a painful childhood, current adverse events, and/or chronically devaluing social messages (Brach, 2003; Briere, 2014). It also includes the notion that everyone, even the client, deserves to be happy and not be maltreated (as one client put it, "why not? Why don't I deserve what everyone should get?"). In this regard, investigation of the basis for one's triggered responses, whether through ReGAIN or more broadly in therapy, works to debunk the myth of intrinsic badness (Briere, 1989) by uncovering other, more accurate and self-compassionate, reasons for upsetting thoughts, intrusive phenomena, and problematic behavior, and by exploring one's basic entitlement to well-being.

- *Nonidentify* **with triggered thoughts, feelings, and memories.** This final step often arises in response to previous steps (Brach, 2013), especially the metacognitive aspects of *Investigation*. From a Western, self-oriented perspective, *nonidentification* refers to one of the fruits of mindfulness and metacognitive awareness: the realization that who we are is not defined by our emotions, thoughts, or memories; we receive our internal experiences, but to some extent we exist separately from them. As one Buddhist teacher notes, summarizing from other Buddhist and Hindu writers, "You are not your thoughts; you are the observer of your thoughts" (Ray, 2015).

Nonidentification is inherent in the metacognitive self-talk described in Chapter 5. For example:

- "Just because I think/feel it doesn't mean it's true."
- "These are just thoughts, not facts."
- "I am not defined by my history or how people judge me."
- "I feel _____ but these are just feelings, they aren't who I am."
- "I am not my thoughts."
- "Although I feel angry/bad/unlovable right now, that doesn't mean that I am an angry/bad/unlovable person."

- In the context of ReGAIN for triggered states, this skill involves metacognitively not identifying with activated internal experiences, especially those that suggest intrinsic badness or undeservingness. For example, a client might be able to say, "Just because I was raped as a kid doesn't mean that I am a lifelong victim, or that I deserve for people to treat me badly. I am not my history. Even though I sometimes blame myself, rape was what was done to me; it doesn't have anything to do with who I really am."

Brach's New RAIN Model

Since 2013, Tara Brach has replaced the *Nonidentify* step of RAIN with *Nurture with self-compassion*. She notes, "We've found that the RAIN process is more transformative when N-Nurture is intentionally engaged as a full step on its own" (*www.tarabrach.com/rain/#rainchange*). In Brach's revised version, *Nonidentify* is not considered an active step; instead, it occurs "after the RAIN," when the individual comes to recognize that her identity is not confined to any specific pattern of emotions or thoughts.

An Example of ReGAINing

Taken together, the components of ReGAIN allow the client to address triggered states directly in a concrete, structured way, and, thereby, may be useful in reducing the probability of a DRB. In the following example, Zoie works her way through the ReGAIN procedure following a perceived rejection.

> Zoie is a 21-year-old woman who has been in RA-focused psychotherapy for 2 years, following an episode of self-injury that was misinterpreted as a suicide attempt, prompting a brief psychiatric hospitalization. She has spent considerable time in treatment processing her abandonment at age 5 by her drug-addicted mother, and long-term psychological abuse and neglect by her grandmother. She is learning to identify and manage her easily triggered feelings of emptiness and self-hatred. In response, Zoie's self-injurious behavior has decreased, as has, to a lesser extent, her tendency to feel rejected and devalued in relationships. At her therapist's suggestion, she attended a mindfulness course and has since successfully used the ReGAIN tool on several occasions to forestall episodes of self-injury.
>
> After a childhood friend seemingly terminated their 15-year relationship during a heated argument, Zoie is again feeling compelled to hurt herself. Although their friendship has always been intense and labile, and it is likely that this breach, too, will resolve over time, her friend was especially harsh in her

condemnation of Zoie, saying things she didn't really mean but that were triggering to Zoie. Zoie was able to get an appointment with her therapist for the late afternoon, but she is currently overwhelmed by anger, shame, and a strong desire to cut herself. As she has in the past, she turns to ReGAIN, moving in and out of sequence, sometimes circling back to an earlier step, then jumping to a later one.

Recognition

- "I can't believe she said those things. I hate her! I can't believe I let her be my friend! She's right, I'm stupid and disgusting. I so need to hurt myself right now. She was my best friend!"
- "Oh my God, I am so messed up. I am so triggered. I have to get out of this. I don't want to cut myself. I'm triggered, this isn't real."
- "OK, it's too real; she said those things. But this is way over the top. I gotta ReGAIN this, because I'm overreacting."

Grounding

- "OK, deep breath. Nice and slow. I'm OK, some of this is just the past, I'm just triggered. That was then, this is now."
- "No, why did she say that I'm a _____? She's the _____!"
- "OK, noticing the room, my feet on the floor. Let it in, let it out. Do a little mindfulness, watch my thoughts and feelings come and go. I'm fine. Think about [her therapist]. What would she say? She'd say I am OK. I'm OK."

Allowing and Self-Compassion

- "I'm not overreacting, this is just what happens when I get triggered. I have to stay with this, stay with these feelings. I need to breathe, like [her therapist] taught me. Just let myself be sad and mad."
- "No, it hurts too much, she was my best friend. I loved her, and she treated me like [expletive]."
- "OK, breathing, follow the breath. Just let it be, it always gets better when you just let it be. It's OK to hate her, because it's just how I feel right now, and I don't really. She probably doesn't hate me either, she's done this before. I just need to hold myself and cry."
- "Just let it be, I'm sad, and that makes perfect sense. I'm a good person, not bad, these are just thoughts that she's right and I suck."
- "I need to give myself a break. This is hard, but I'm handling it OK. It's sad that I have to keep feeling this way whenever someone hurts me, but it's not my fault, and I can handle it."

- "OK, allowing, allowing."
- "But I need to allow myself to cut myself. Because I'm a disgusting mess nobody loves. Not true, just triggered thoughts. It's OK to have the thought, it's normal and fine. But just let the thoughts be there, don't act on them. Just surf the urge, let it rise and let it fall away. Easy to say. Breathe. I am upset and hurt, that's all this is. I am a good person who deserves to be happy."

Investigation

- "This is so familiar. Like with my grandmother. Calling me names and putting me down. My mom leaving me alone."
- "Here we go again, I'm a broken record, just treat me like [expletive] and it's pity-party time."
- "Pity party? Where did that come from? Those aren't my words. OK, that's Grandma talking, that I need to take stock of myself. Stock of myself? Those aren't my words either. I'm just so upset. But I get to be upset."
- "I hate her! She said I am a loser that nobody likes! No wonder I'm triggered. Hello, Grandma."
- "I don't really hate her. She was mean, but I said things, too. I think we both were reliving the past. She certainly was hurt by her dad. And she's hurt now, too. I hope she's OK. Trigger, trigger. OK, this is working a little, I'm not in the past, I'm right here. I have friends, and a good job, and a good therapist."

Nonidentification

- "I know this place. I feel like the abused and unloved little girl I used to be. But that's not true anymore. That time has passed. I'm just triggered. I'm not unlovable. Thoughts are just thoughts, and when they get like this, they're usually wrong. These are just thoughts and feelings, not anything more."
- "This will work out. I'm still me and I can handle this. I'm feeling hurt and upset, but I am who I am, a good person, who has done a lot of work on herself. This is just the drama of life, plus a little help from my past. And [her friend]. And Grandma. This will pass. It has before. I hope she's OK."

CHAPTER 8

Processing Trauma- and Attachment-Related Memories

Anna is a 47-year-old woman who has been in therapy for 8 months following a sexual assault by a coworker. In her intake interview. Anna reported symptoms of posttraumatic stress and depression, and described instances of self-cutting—behavior that she engaged in briefly as an adolescent and that has now reemerged. With reluctance, she also disclosed a history of severe neglect and sexual abuse when she was young, although she attributed her current difficulties exclusively to the recent assault.

Given Anna's posttraumatic stress, her therapist began treatment with prolonged exposure (PE). This involved having Anna describe the sexual assault in detail, often in the first-person, present tense, for 45 minutes at a time. Almost immediately, however, her self-injurious behavior escalated, and her responses to the therapist became increasingly angry. In response, the clinician terminated PE and focused more on stabilization and emotional regulation techniques. Upon further discussion with Anna, it became clear that trigger chaining was an issue: Memories of the recent assault were activating memories of childhood abuse, and her therapist's behaviors, although benign, were inadvertently triggering attachment-level cognitive schema involving disattunement and abandonment.

With a greater focus on stabilization and emotional regulation, and attention to the impact of her attachment history on the current therapeutic relationship, Anna's self-injury has diminished substantially, and her connection with her therapist has improved. Currently, her therapy involves a more titrated, client-guided approach to therapeutic exposure, for example, moving from memories of her recent assault to a brief relaxation exercise, then to careful exploration of memories of childhood abuse and neglect, followed by a grounding exercise, then back to the assault or another trauma. Importantly, both she and her therapist work to ensure that exposure-related distress does not overwhelm her compromised, but growing, emotional regulation skills.

Most existing approaches to avoidance behaviors such as DRBs or excessive substance use (e.g., DBT, interpersonal psychotherapy [IPT], MBRP, and *Seeking Safety*) focus primarily on emotional regulation training, mindfulness, and coping and interpersonal skills development, and provide, at best, only informal (Linehan, 1993) therapeutic exposure. In contrast, RA-focused therapy specifically includes a range of interventions that support emotional processing of the trauma- and attachment-related memories that contribute to DRBs.

It is understandable that some therapies are less concerned with therapeutic exposure in work with DRB-involved clients. First, such clients are especially likely to come to treatment in a state of relative instability and dysregulation, and therefore require more immediate interventions that increase their safety, stabilize their internal environment, and help them deal with potentially overwhelming intrusive experiences. Second, especially for those with major childhood trauma and/or attachment disturbance, ill-timed or less titrated therapeutic exposure can challenge stability and coping capacities, and potentially lead to overwhelming emotional states and experiences, if not premature termination.

Apropos of the latter concern, the average therapy completion rate (often defined as attending more than six sessions of an evidence-based treatment) in real-world clinical contexts is often less than 50% (e.g., Mott et al., 2014; Watts et al., 2014; see a detailed review by Najavits, 2015). Drop-out during exposure therapy may be even more common for the individuals most relevant to this book, for example those suffering from substance abuse, depression, dissociation, suicidality, more severe posttraumatic stress, and, especially, borderline personality disorder (e.g., Zayfert & Black, 2000; Zayfert et al., 2005).

This is a well-known conundrum for those who work with complex trauma survivors, especially those engaged in DRBs: Therapeutic exposure to trauma memories clearly can be helpful to the extent that it addresses the underlying basis for the client's avoidance. Yet it can be problematic if, for whatever reason, the client is unable to tolerate the distress associated with activated memories, and develops more symptoms or drops out of treatment. This issue—whether and when to directly address trauma memories in therapy—is currently a source of fruitful discussion in the trauma literature, with some writers suggesting a primary focus on building stability, coping responses, interpersonal relationships, and emotional regulation capacities (e.g., Linehan, 1993; Markowitz et al., 2015; Najavits, 2002; although see Najavits & Johnson, 2014), others emphasizing the benefit of therapeutic exposure to trauma memories (e.g., Foa et al., 2007; Zoellner et al., 2011), and still others asserting the importance of both, albeit typically focusing on capacity and skills development before memory processing (e.g., Bohus et al., 2013; Cloitre et al., 2006).

The RA perspective holds that within the context of a positive therapeutic relationship, a combination of stabilization, emotional regulation training (including trigger management), and titrated processing of distressing memories is likely to be most effective in work with those prone to DRBs. It may even be misleading to view these aspects of therapy as independent of one another. The positive effects of a good therapeutic relationship, for example, may include activation and processing of childhood memories, reworking of negative attachment-level assumptions about self and others, and development of a more robust emotional regulation repertoire. Similarly, therapeutic exposure to traumatic memories typically requires a safe and supportive relationship, metacognitive acceptance of current internal experiences, and some level of emotional regulation capacity.

In fact, although not always described as such, even mindfulness and emotional regulation interventions can lead to therapeutic exposure. To the extent that such activities result in decreased avoidance, they naturally allow emotional processing of previously avoided memories. In this sense, it may be a bit of a "straw person" debate as to whether exposure should be part of therapy. The issue instead is how exposure is conducted, and whether it can be done in ways that are safe, that do not overwhelm, and that meaningfully address the underlying etiologies of DRBs.

RA-focused treatment takes advantage of these exposure opportunities whenever possible, because it is unlikely that the interventions described in the previous chapters will, in and of themselves, completely eliminate DRBs. In most cases, even if the client is able to regulate his emotional responses to trauma, and learn ways to manage triggered responses, the underlying association between trauma stimuli and painful thoughts and feelings still exists, and can continue to produce distress. Although a major benefit for DRB-involved people, emotion regulation and tolerance skills do not especially address the actual trauma or attachment memories; they primarily ameliorate triggered effects of memory in the moment.

For this reason, an RA perspective focuses on both sides of the DRB equation: first working to increase resilience to triggered states, then carefully addressing the memories behind these states. Fortunately, these two foci often work together: (1) Increasing emotional regulation capacity reduces the need for avoidance, thereby allowing exposure to previously overwhelming memories, and (2) repeated titrated exposure to painful memories can increase emotional tolerance, as the client "gets used to" distress that he previously avoided. As noted by Najavits (2013)

> The goal is thus to move beyond the extremes that have historically guided therapy of PTSD/SUD [substance use disorder] clients: either none should do past-focused work ("they are too fragile") or all should do it ("it's helpful for everyone"). The clinician's task is to balance these opposites, focusing on how, when, and whether to move in and out of the work with each client. (p. 6)

This chapter reviews ways in which the client can directly process trauma- and attachment-related memories so that they are less able to motivate DRBs. Because some of the ideas in the RA approach differ from other treatment paradigms, we first explore several constructs integral to this model.

Emotional Processing

The term *therapeutic exposure* is used in this book to refer to a process in which the client is asked to talk about (and, thus, remember) past traumatic events in the specific context of a safe and caring therapeutic environment. As will be discussed, when exposure occurs in safety and with therapeutic support, trauma and attachment memories can slowly lose their power to produce distress, thereby reducing the motivation for DRBs. When this occurs, the client's activation–regulation balance can move toward equilibrium, in part due to increased emotional regulation capacity, but also decreased activatable distress. Although titrated exposure and activation is described in detail later in this chapter, it is best understood as part of a larger phenomenon, generally referred to as emotional processing.

PE, Fear Structures, and Trauma Schemas

Emotional processing was defined by Foa and Kozak (1986) as a process whereby erroneous trauma-related perceptions, beliefs, and expectations (what they call "pathological fear structures") are activated and are, through habituation, modified or replaced by new information. The basic idea of exposure-based habituation is that the client is repeatedly triggered into this fear structure, then "stays with" this state for relatively long periods of time (often up to 90 minutes per session [Foa & Rothbaum, 1998], hence the term *prolonged* exposure), until the emotion dissipates (habituates). *Successful habituation* is often defined as a reduction in subjective units of distress of at least 50% within a given session (e.g., Foa, Yadin, & Lichner, 2012).

Although habituation of fear has been a central goal of PE, other cognitive–emotional states are also associated with trauma-related stimuli, including anger, shame, humiliation, self-hatred, helplessness, and abandonment preoccupation—none of which are specifically targeted by classic exposure therapy (Linehan, 1993). The term *trauma schema* is used here for these more complex internal phenomena, defined here as systems of interlinked (*chained*) trauma- or attachment-related memories, beliefs, expectations, and emotions that can be triggered by reminiscent stimuli. Interestingly, it is likely that, despite its initial focus on fear, therapeutic exposure also, to some extent, reduces nonanxiety-related symptoms (O'Donohue & Fisher, 2012). Clinical experience suggests that memory activation, nonreinforcement, emotional processing, correction of erroneous beliefs, and counterconditioning all occur in the treatment of these phenomena, as well as fear, and research on exposure-based treatments often reveal reductions in a range of PTSD symptoms, anger, guilt, and depression, as well as anxiety (e.g., Cahill, Rauch, Hembree, & Foa, 2003; Foa et al., 2005).

Beyond Habituation

As opposed to Foa and Kozak (1986), the RA model is not habituation-focused. In fact, the habituation construct has lost much of its favor in the psychological literature, largely because the outcome of exposure therapy does not actually appear to be affected by whether fear habituates within—or sometimes even across—sessions (e.g., Baker et al., 2010; Prenoveau, Craske, Liao, & Ornitz, 2013; van Minnen & Foa, 2006). In the absence of habituation as an active ingredient, an obvious question arises: Is it necessary to have prolonged exposure to a specific triggered cognitive–emotional state or fear structure in order for processing to occur?

Recent research suggests that it may not. Several studies have shown that less sustained exposure to trauma memories is just as effective as classical PE in reducing posttraumatic stress (e.g., Nacasch et al., 2015; van Minnen & Foa, 2006; Sloan, Marx, Lee, & Resick, 2018), leading Foa and McLean (2016) to conclude that "the fact that within-session fear reduction does not predict treatment outcome suggests that the length of PE sessions can be shortened without compromising efficacy" (p. 11).

In fact, recent work suggests that exposure may not even be necessary for symptom reduction. Markowitz and colleagues (2015) found that IPT (Weissman, Markowitz, & Klerman, 2000), which does not involve exposure or habituation, was at least equivalent to PE in reducing symptoms of PTSD, and was more effective in treating comorbid depression. Similarly, other therapies—for example, cognitive processing therapy (CPT; Resick & Schnicke, 1992), eye movement desensitization and reprocessing (EMDR; Shapiro, 1991, 2017), written exposure therapy (WET; Sloan et al., 2018), and Seeking Safety (Najavits, 2002)—have demonstrated efficacy in treating PTSD without obvious habituation components. The existence of these other effective therapies does not negate the usefulness of PE in all instances(e.g., Peck, Schumacher, Stasiewicz, & Coffey, 2018), but it does suggest that, especially for DRB-involved clients with low emotional regulation and distress intolerance, there may be effective alternatives to habituation-based—and therefore prolonged—exposure approaches.

Inhibitory Learning

To add to the complexity, it is becoming clear that exposure-based extinction does not actually involve the deletion or erasure of the association between a triggering stimulus and a conditioned (e.g., trauma-related) response. Indeed, these associations appear to remain in memory, even if they are no longer called upon (Bjork & Bjork, 1992). As Jacoby and Abramowitz (2016) note, "Once they are learned, such associations don't fade over time; rather access to them does" (p. 30). The continuing presence of old learning may explain in part why some extinguished associations are susceptible to spontaneous recovery after treatment. Such "relapses" of symptomatology appear to be more likely in situations or contexts that are different from those under which extinction learning originally occurred, and when additional traumatization or danger occurs after treatment, refreshing old trauma-related associations (Craske et al., 2014).

The continuing presence of old memories aside newer versions of them is a central focus of *inhibitory learning theory* (Lang, Craske, & Bjork, 1999), a perspective that has growing acceptance (Jacoby & Abramowitz, 2016). It suggests that therapy-based learning—for example, that interpersonal vulnerability does not always lead to danger—must compete with "old" but still potentially available expectancies (e.g., those formed in the context of childhood abuse). The difference between inhibitory learning and earlier habituation perspectives has significant implications for trauma and attachment processing, as described later in this chapter.

Counterconditioning

An RA approach to memory processing also includes significant attention to counterconditioning, to some extent as originally proposed decades ago in Wolpe's (1969) systematic desensitization approach. Wolpe hypothesized that if an anxiety-evoking stimulus (e.g., a trigger) is repeatedly presented while the person is in an anxiety-incompatible state, the association between the trigger and the anxiety responses will weaken. Interestingly, recent research (e.g., Högberg & Hällström, 2018; Lane, Ryan, Nadel, & Greenberg, 2014; Nadel, Hupbach, Gomez, & Newman-Smith, 2012) offers some support for Wolpe's contention, primarily in terms of what is described as *memory reconsolidation* in the next section. Translated into an RA perspective, counterconditioning is likely to occur when the client reexperiences trauma- or attachment-related memories in the context of a compassionate and caring therapeutic relationship, or when therapeutic activities such as relaxation or mindfulness training are integrated into therapeutic exposure, such that the memory at least partially changes its valence and loses some of its ability to produce distress upon being triggered.

Reconsolidation

Recent research may explain how memory inhibition and counterconditioning effects actually reduce triggerable emotional distress during successful emotional processing. Studies suggests that there is a golden window of several hours following the activation of a memory, during which time it can be updated with new information or altered emotionality, then "reconsolidated" back into the brain as a newer, more powerful memory (e.g., Tronson & Taylor, 2007). In this regard, Lane and colleagues (2015) propose that "the essential ingredients of therapeutic change include: (1) reactivating old memories; [and] (2) engaging in new emotional experiences that are incorporated into these reactivated memories via the process of reconsolidation" (p. 1). As noted by Högberg and Hällström (2018), this process "means that an autobiographical memory, when activated, can change its emotional valence in a short time frame and be reconsolidated with new emotional valence as part of personal memory" (p. 2). From this perspective, if a client can access distress-incompatible states (e.g., relaxation, warm feelings associated with a good therapeutic relationship)—or insights that decrease distress—during and soon after a painful memory is activated, future triggering of this updated and reconsolidated memory will be less associated with negative emotional states.

Thus, RA-focused therapy relies heavily on the counterconditioning and distress-reducing aspects of the therapeutic relationship, and often intersperses exposure with periods of relaxation or mindfulness, less distressing activities, such as psychoeducation, present-centered discussions, or emotion regulation practice. In contrast, exposure that is excessively prolonged or potentially overwhelming, and does not include the elicitation of positive or calming states, might theoretically lead to reconsolidation of structures and schemas that contain even more distress.

The option of counterconditioning trauma or attachment memories seemingly brings the therapeutic relationship into cognitive-behavioral approaches to trauma therapy. As is described later, it also suggests the importance of attachment in some instances of trauma processing, since the positive feelings associated with a caring therapeutic relationship may involve, in part, the activation of attachment-related neurobiology.

Memory Targets

In most exposure-based trauma treatments, the client is asked to choose her "worst" or most significant trauma memory, so that it can be elicited and habituated over a number of sessions. Following habituation-based processing of this memory, another memory may be chosen. An RA-focused perspective, on the other hand, does not constrain treatment to one trauma at a time, for several reasons.

First, as noted, recent research suggests that habituation is probably irrelevant to positive treatment outcomes. As a result, there is no specific reason why one memory must be habituated before another is considered. In fact, research has not yet demonstrated an optimal exposure period for clinical efficacy, although increasingly shorter exposure intervals appear to yield equivalent outcomes, and no research indicates that multiple, more brief, exposures to different memories are inferior to longer exposures that focus on a single memory. Furthermore, as noted earlier, inhibitory learning may be more effective when trauma-based associations are elicited and processed in a variety of different contexts and points in time.

Second, DRB-involved clients typically have a history of many trauma exposures and attachment breaches; thus, it can be difficult to pick "the worst" trauma- or attachment-related memory. Were that even possible, a number of other traumas of nearly the same severity would seemingly go untreated.

In fact, exposure to a single trauma memory is likely impossible in the first place. Especially in complex trauma survivors, exposure to one memory often activates recollections of other traumas and/or attachment breaches and their cognitive–emotional sequels, leading to a chained cascade of internal associations and activated states described in this book as trigger chaining. For example, a person might be processing memories of a sexual assault in therapy, which then trigger shame and self-blame associated with memories of child sexual abuse, which then activate early, largely implicit memories of neglect or caretaker disengagement, causing the client to feel sudden distrust of the therapist. In such situations, it would not be accurate to say that a single trauma memory was being processed.

Given this complexity, clinical experience suggests that therapy may be most helpful when clients are able to determine which trauma they want to address at any specific moment in treatment, rather than being refocused on the originally agreed-upon therapeutic target. Because trauma memories tend to activate one another through trigger chaining, and most posttraumatic stress disorders appear to arise from multiple (not single) traumas, the RA model therapist generally follows the client from one memory to the next within a single session, gently encouraging some level of processing in each instance, and making sure that the client does not flood himself with too many memories over a short period of time. For example, the client might begin the session discussing an episode of child abuse, then move on to a rape experience in adolescence, and later describe a paramedic's judgmental comments after a recent overdose. In each instance, the therapist would encourage her to verbalize the event in as much detail as possible without the process being overwhelming. The therapist would also provide visible support and validation regarding the experiences, checking in with the client as to her current feelings and associations, and perhaps suggesting a brief relaxation or mindfulness exercise.

Not only should the client be able to determine which trauma she wants to address at any moment in treatment, the habituation data also suggest that the exposure process need not be extended nor extreme. Instead, such activities may be most tolerable when they are under the client's control as well. As noted by Linehan (1993), such personal control "may itself be therapeutic and render future exposure less frightening" (p. 352).

Self-Titration

The therapist's willingness to follow the client from memory to memory, and allow him to determine the extent and intensity of exposure, does not mean that instances of client memory avoidance are ignored (Constance Dalenberg, personal communication, February 25, 2018). Instead, the therapist might note at some point in time the client's earlier movement from one memory or topic to another, at which point a nonjudgmental discussion might ensue as to the reasons underlying such switching. If the movement was due to memories triggering memories (trigger chaining), repeated consideration of this process may increase the client's metacognitive appreciation of triggering phenomena, per se. If the switch was in the service of reduced activation, this response would be discussed as well, generally in terms of distress titration. In the latter instance, two questions might be asked: Why was avoidance necessary at that moment in time, and would less avoidance be possible the next time? Notably, these questions are predicated on the idea that avoidance is neither intrinsically "bad" nor is it a sign that the client is resisting therapy, but rather that it is a coping strategy that has upsides and downsides, the magnitude and balance of which vary from moment to moment.

The Efficiency of Multiple Targets

Although multitarget processing might appear to be less efficient than extended attention to a single memory, in practice, most DRB-involved clients have been exposed to multiple traumas and attachment disruptions in their lives that, cumulatively, better predict posttraumatic outcomes than do single-event traumas. In such instances, multitarget processing is likely to be more helpful than engaging in a series of separate, extended exposure interventions for each of a large number of distressing memories. Furthermore, clinical experience suggests that when the reasons for exposure are made clear to clients, and they are allowed to choose which memory to focus on at any specific moment, they often end up returning to the most problematic or distress-producing memories over time. In this way, greater exposure to significant traumas typically still occurs, but these memories emerge naturally, based on which memory especially draw the client's attention or intrudes to the greatest extent during treatment, and the client's self-determination is honored and reinforced.

Another benefit of multiple targets and variable levels of exposure is predicted by inhibitory learning theory. Specifically, it may be possible to increase the chances that therapy-based trauma processing will persist and continue to override or inhibit earlier abuse-related emotional associations, so that treatment effects are more durable and generalized. Although Craske et al. (2014) list a variety of techniques, two seem especially relevant to trauma treatment. Specifically, new learning may be strengthened when therapy:

- *Highlights expectancy violations.* This occurs when the client is encouraged to discuss his expectations of what will happen if he talks about the trauma, feels the attendant feelings, opens up to relationships, avoids employing a DRB, or tries new things that contradict trauma-related learning. When this is paired with evidence that the client's expectations turned out to be incorrect, the disparity should be gently highlighted in subsequent discussions. In other words, as noted by Craske et al. (2014), the more the expectancy can be violated by experience, the less trauma-related conditioned responses are available for triggering. The wide-ranging targets of RA-guided treatment typically mean that multiple schema and fear structures are activated and processed; hence, multiple expectancies are contradicted and counterconditioned by the safety and support of the therapeutic relationship.

- *Involves variable exposures and includes multiple contexts.* As noted earlier, distress extinction is more durable and persistent when memories are processed from a variety of different contexts, perspectives, and situations, and at variable levels of intensity and duration (Craske et al., 2014). RA-focused treatment, by its nature, facilitates inhibitory learning, since it involves repeated titrated exposure to a range of implicit and explicit memories and contexts, often as they interact with, and trigger, one another. Furthermore, depending on the client's immediate activation–regulation status, titrated exposure varies in intensity and duration over time, thereby deepening the unavailability of past learning. As well, trauma-related associations are addressed both verbally and through relational processing, providing different "angles" and approaches to trauma-conditioned responses.

Interspersal

As noted in the counterconditioning and consolidation discussions, an important aspect of RA-oriented exposure exercises is the use of relaxation, mindfulness, nondistressing discussions, and positive relational activation, which are *interspersed* between periods of exposure. For example, the client might be invited to use a mindfulness meditation exercise like the ones in Appendix 1, then engage in a brief (e.g., 10–20 minute) period of titrated exposure to a memory of child abuse, perhaps followed by more mindfulness or a relaxation exercise, and then another brief exposure and further relaxation.

Interestingly, this approach is to some extent contrary to classic exposure models. The developers of PE, for example, specifically discourage the use of breath exercises during exposure because "we want them to experience their ability to cope with trauma-related memories and situations without special devices" (Foa et al., 2007, p. 2). Their concerns likely relate to research suggesting that the use of "safety" activities (behaviors that allay fear during exposure) sometimes reduces the effectiveness of therapeutic exposure (Helbig-Lang & Petermann, 2010; Weisman & Rodebaugh, 2018). However, others have not found evidence of adverse safety effects (e.g., Deacon et al., 2010; Meulders, Van Daele, Volders, & Vlaeyen, 2016), and some writers (e.g., Meulders et al., 2016) suggest that safety behaviors may actually increase the tolerability of exposure and support the client's sense of self-efficacy. Ultimately, however, these studies have limited implications for interspersal, since it does not occur during exposure episodes, but rather before and after them. As a result, rather than potentially inhibiting the effects of exposure, interspersal may facilitate emotional processing by pairing adversity-related memories with distress-reducing states, which then may be reconsolidated in a less activating form.

Perhaps more immediately relevant to concerns about attenuating the effects of therapeutic exposure, recent research indicates that prior mindfulness exercises do not negate the effectiveness of subsequent exposure (e.g., Treanor, 2011) and may have neuropsychological effects that facilitate recovery from posttraumatic stress (King et al., 2016). In support of this research, Treanor (2011) outlines, in an extensive review, a variety of ways in which mindfulness prior to exposure may enhance extinction learning and thereby facilitate exposure effects. Research also does not indicate that prior relaxation interferes with the effects of exposure, although most studies suggest that it does not add to exposure in reducing anxiety-related symptoms (Tyron, 2005). However, in a study of clients more similar to those engaged in DRBs, Cloitre et al. (2002) found that a positive therapeutic relationship and the development of emotional regulation skills prior to emotional processing increased the effectiveness of subsequent therapeutic exposure activities.

There are also little data suggesting that *post*-exposure relaxation is problematic and good reason to suggest that it might be helpful in reducing unresolved exposure-related distress (e.g., Peck Schumacher, Stasiewicz, & Coffey, 2018). Deescalation of triggered memory effects may be especially relevant to DRB-involved clients, who otherwise might respond to continuing distress with postsession avoidance such as self-injury or substance abuse.

An additional potential benefit of interspersal is its tendency to constrain the intensity of emotional activation during therapeutic exposure. By alternating periods of arousal with activities that down-regulate arousal, memories of trauma- or attachment-related distress have fewer chances to build to extreme levels; thus, the client is provided with the opportunity to move in and out of memory activation without feeling overwhelmed. And when triggered, nonoverwhelming emotional distress is subsequently downregulated, it is more likely that the reconsolidated memory will contain less negative emotional valence. Not only is this a form of titrated exposure, it may, as noted more generally by Linehan (1993) and Meulders et al. (2016), decrease the DRB-involved client's fear of exposure and increase his sense of control and self-efficacy.

Finally, interspersal provides the client with multiple opportunities to learn and practice coping responses to moderate—but not overwhelming—arousal in relative safety, and thereby develop a broader repertoire of emotional regulation skills. As the client is repeatedly exposed to "handleable" levels of conditioned emotional distress, she is able to experiment with different emotional regulation approaches, as well as slowly developing greater tolerance to triggered emotional distress (Briere, 2002a).

Summary: RA-Focused Trauma Processing

Based on the preceding discussion, the RA model holds that trauma processing occurs when exposure to trauma-reminiscent stimuli triggers emotional, cognitive, and sensory memories, some of which are explicit and others of which are implicit, yet

- these activated memories are not reinforced by danger or rejection in the session.
- the client is free to choose which memories to process and for how long.
- memory processing does not exceed the client's emotional regulation capacities, and therefore is not experienced as overwhelming.
- activated memories are counterconditioned by opposite emotional experiences and new information, generally arising from positive aspects of the therapeutic relationship, new insights, and previously learned relaxation, grounding, and/or mindfulness exercises.

This process, in turn, ideally leads to

- The development of new schemas that contradict existing trauma-related beliefs.
- Inhibition of previously conditioned associations between trauma-reminiscent stimuli and painful emotional responses.
- Subsequent reconsolidation of the traumatic memories, albeit now with new information (e.g., more affirming and accurate schemas), less conditioned emotional distress, and the positive effects of therapist compassion and caring.
- Less distress upon future memory activation, leading to decreased need to engage in DRBs.

Processing Explicit and Implicit Memories

Up to this point, trauma memory processing has been described in general terms. Yet the two major types of memories (implicit and explicit) vary significantly according to what they contain, how they are encoded, and how they are experienced once triggered. These differences have significant implications for how each is processed.

Explicit Memory

As described in Chapter 3, explicit memory is generally verbally mediated, autobiographical, and subject to intentional recall. This type of memory is often called *episodic,* in that it involves recollection of life events, including trauma. An explicit memory of a traumatic event might include, for example, information on where one was assaulted, who was involved, and when it occurred. Explicit memory typically requires language (Byrne, 2017), and a sufficiently developed sense of self (Bauer & Fivush, 2010); thus, it generally first appears developmentally around ages 2–3. A noteworthy aspect of such memories is that they are recognized as such: Access to explicit memories includes awareness that one is remembering.

Implicit Memory

As discussed, implicit memories can influence behavior but cannot be voluntarily recalled, and are therefore sometimes considered to be "unconscious" (Greenwald & Banaji, 2017). Implicit memories of trauma and attachment history are nonverbal in nature; often sensory or emotional, but sometimes cognitive; nonautobiographical; and often easily triggered by reminiscent stimuli. Such memories do not come with information that they are memories; when triggered, they often appear as perceptions or experiences in the here and now. A classic example of a triggered implicit memory is a flashback, in which a triggered sensory memory of a past trauma is "relived" as if it involved a present event.

Whether a given memory is explicit or implicit depends on when in life it was encoded and the level of distress or arousal present at the time it occurred. Memories that are largely implicit commonly occur under two conditions: in early childhood, prior to the onset of language (Schore, 2000), and under highly stressful conditions, when brain systems associated with explicit memory (especially the hippocampus) are less functional but other systems involved in high threat situations (especially the amygdala) are strongly activated (Metcalfe & Jacobs, 1998). Implicit encoding may predominate in other situations as well, however, for example, when someone experiences a trauma under the influence of alcohol (White, 2003) or a date rape drug such as Rohypnol or Versed (Stewart, Buffett-Jerrott, Finley, Wright, & Valois Gomez, 2006), or explicit memory of an event has been compromised by dementia (Harrison, Son, Kim, & Whall, 2007).

Perhaps not surprisingly, trauma processing is to some extent more focused on implicit than on explicit memories. Many of the symptoms of posttraumatic stress (e.g., flashbacks, nightmares, and autonomic nervous system reactivity in response to trauma cues) are implicit in nature, as are emotional responses and schemas that are conditioned to trauma-related stimuli and emerge when triggered.

Even more critically, early attachment-related memories involving caretaker emotional unavailability, loss, neglect, threat, or ambivalence are, by definition, implicit, since the child has yet to develop the language and neurobiology necessary for explicit memory encoding. Consistent with the implicit memory literature, insecure attachment phenomena operate outside of conscious awareness and, when triggered, can result in the emergence of archaic thoughts, feelings, sensations, and behaviors that are nevertheless experienced as current, contemporaneous phenomena.

This is not to say that explicit memory processing is irrelevant to trauma treatment. Autobiographically encoded memories, when remembered, also can result in great distress. Not only do they contain verbally mediated information on the hurtful event(s) that are linked to emotional pain, the inferences the client forms upon being victimized may be encoded in explicit memory as potentially distorted systems of meaning, negative self- or other evaluations, or fearful expectations about the future. Similarly, crying when remembering a recently lost loved one, for example, or becoming angry when thinking about an interpersonal slight, are often in response to explicit memory phenomena.

Explicit-to-Implicit Triggering

Not only can explicit memories cause distress, but they can also be triggers for implicit memory activation. In fact, much of the therapeutic exposure process involves the use of explicit memory to trigger implicit memory (Briere & Scott, 2014). For example, requests that a client talk about her trauma is a request for her to access autobiographical memory, which, when engaged, offers a rich source of triggers for implicit trauma schema and fear structures. When these cognitions and emotions are repeatedly activated in a safe environment, but not reinforced, extinction can occur. For example:

> Frank is talking to his therapist about being bullied as a child at school. As he describes being pushed to the ground, kicked, hit, and exposed to homophobic taunts and threats, he becomes increasingly upset and appears to be reliving the experience. From a technical perspective, Frank has described this trauma in sufficient detail that some level of context reinstatement is occurring: His autobiographical memories have become reminiscent stimuli that are triggering implicit memories of fear, anger, and shame, encoded at the time of the trauma. His sudden distress is not in response to memory; it *is* the memory.
>
> As he repeatedly describes what happened to him, across sessions, it is likely that Frank's trauma-related distress will go unreinforced in the absence of current danger, and will be counterconditioned by therapeutic attention, caring, and support. Notably, his explicit memories of the bullying will not decrease: They may even become more accurate and detailed with further therapeutic exploration. What will typically lessen is the capacity of stimuli reminiscent of bullying to activate implicitly encoded emotional pain. Frank may still be angry about what was done to him, but this anger is more likely to be a contextually relevant response to explicit memory, not implicit reliving of the past.

Implicit Triggering Alone

Not all triggers of implicit memory are explicit. In many cases, the individual will encounter stimuli in the environment—especially in relational contexts—that directly trigger implicit recollections. In such cases, autobiographical memory may be absent or to some extent irrelevant. This direct triggering is associated with a considerable amount of suffering among those with histories of difficult attachment experiences or child maltreatment. For example, someone who feels rejected by a friend or lover may be triggered into intense feelings of abandonment and unlovability that, when overwhelming, may require an avoidance response. In this regard, most "impulsive" or "acting-out" behaviors are likely the result of implicit triggering.

Fortunately, the tendency for implicit memories to be triggered by reminiscent stimuli can be taken advantage of in the therapy session. As described below, therapy for attachment disturbance and/or early childhood trauma often involves the client forming a relationship with the therapist that contains a multitude of potential triggers—whether increased emotional intimacy, therapist characteristics that are in some way similar to the client's caretaker(s), or aspects of the therapeutic relationship that tend to activate unaddressed attachment needs. In such contexts, the client may be triggered into painful, childhood-era emotional states but, at the same time, experience positive feelings associated with the therapeutic relationship. As a result, the client will encounter a lack of agreement between triggered emotions and assumptions and what is actually present in the current environment, potentially leading to counterconditioning, extinction, and decreased triggerability.

Processing Implicit Activations *In Vivo*

Not only can implicit memories be counterconditioned by the therapeutic relationship, they can also be directly processed as they emerge during treatment. As described in Chapter 9, this intervention is often employed later in treatment, however, when it can take advantage of the client's growing metacognitive awareness and emotional regulation capacity.

In vivo processing of implicit memories usually occurs in the context of two phenomena: triggered relational memories and in-session flashbacks. In each case, some aspect of the therapy dialogue or treatment process triggers implicit memories that emerge suddenly; seem out of proportion to the current context; and result in aversive thoughts, emotions, and/or sensations.

In the case of relational activations, for example, the client may suddenly feel abandoned by, or alienated from, the therapist, or experience sudden anger or neediness that she attributes to the clinician's behavior.

Flashbacks, on the other hand, are more sensory intrusions, often experienced as suddenly reliving an instance of abuse or trauma in the session. Unlike relational activations, the client may not attribute what is happening to the therapist, but rather experience a perceptual shift away from the session to the unfolding experiential memory of the trauma. In each case, however, activated distress should not seen as an unfortunate by-product of therapy, or something to talk the client out of, but, rather, as an opportunity to work directly with activated implicit memory.

It is especially important to prepare the client ahead of time (in what is often called *prebriefing* (Briere & Scott, 2014) for *in vivo* processing because she is being asked to consciously discount what her perceptions may be telling her, override source attribution errors, and metacognitively experience the intrusions as implicit memories. For this reason, the rationale for *in vivo* processing should be explained and the client's "buy-in" obtained.

The following are typically the steps of *in vivo* processing of implicit memories:

• After a within-session intrusion of trauma-related negative thoughts or feelings, the client—often with the therapist's assistance—comes to recognize that she is experiencing an activated implicit memory, as opposed to accurately perceiving events in the current moment. This step can be challenging when the activated state is especially powerful (e.g., involving feelings of rejection or abandonment), and it may be that the client can only approximate metacognitive awareness in early attempts. This may mean that the client and clinician need to have multiple discussions about what *seems* real versus what may, in fact, be the true state of affairs at a given moment in therapy. The therapist works to be gentle, nonlecturing, and nondefensive in such dialogues, even when the client strongly disagrees with the therapist about what she is experiencing and believes to be true.

• Following grounding or other stabilizing interventions, if needed, the client is encouraged to sit with, and mindfully "watch," the memory and her reactions to it, exploring with the therapist any associated feelings, thoughts, and sensations. The intent in this stage is to objectify the activated state: studying and discussing it in sufficient depth that its non-real and noncontemporaneous aspects become more obvious. When the client is able to verbalize this lack of correspondence between activation and reality, the disparity is often more clear and the memory is more clearly seen as a memory.

• When appropriate, the client investigates the historical basis for the activated memory, as is done in ReGAINing. In some cases, this will be straightforward. In others, especially if the memory is from early childhood, only a hypothesis can be made, as noted in Chapter 4. Nevertheless, as the client's life history becomes more clear to him, and to the therapist, this guess may be made with greater confidence, although never assumed to be absolute fact. This step can be facilitated by reviewing a previously completed the Triggers-to-Memories Worksheet (Appendix 5).

• The client and therapist further discuss the memory, to the extent it is available, potentially leading to additional exposure and activation. When the actual memory is not available for recall, it may be that further discussion of the flashback or triggered schema will lead to meaningful activation and processing.

The following is an example of a client processing an activated abandonment schema:

CLIENT: Wait. You're just telling me this now? You are going to *Mexico*? I'm sorry I'm having this crisis. It must be very inconvenient for you. When are you going?

THERAPIST: In a month. I'll leave on the 12th and return on the 19th.

CLIENT: Fine. Whatever.

THERAPIST: Hey, Ben, what's going on? You mad at me?

CLIENT: No. Yeah. Actually, I'm really pissed. Here I am, in hell, and you're going off to have margaritas on some beach. Must be nice.

THERAPIST: OK, I get that. I'm sorry my vacation is scheduled for then. Not good. Dr. Green will be my backup for that week.

CLIENT: Right. Like I'd call your substitute shrink.

THERAPIST: Ben, it makes sense that you'd be mad. I'd probably be mad. But I'm wondering, could some of this be triggered? If it is, do you want to work on it, like we talked about before?

[Brief discussion of whether and how the client has been triggered. The therapist stays nondefensive and validates the client's responses, and does not argue or insist that his perceptions are necessarily right. The client slowly concludes that the therapist's upcoming vacation triggers early memories of parental neglect.]

THERAPIST: OK, so, remember, the first step is to stay with how you are feeling. What's it like?

CLIENT: Now it's starting to feel irrational, but I guess I feel like you are really important to me, but I'm not important to you. And that this is a hard time, and you are going away just when I need you.

THERAPIST: Good. Good job, Ben. I mean, I do care about you, but let's go with the feeling right now. What's the biggest part? Do any thoughts or memories come up?

CLIENT: Mostly abandoned . . . And I can feel being really pissed off at you . . . But I know it's not that. My parents didn't give a damn about me. They really didn't. It makes me feel sad. I was just a kid, and I needed them. I remember feeling pretty alone.

[The client continues to describe feelings of early abandonment and parental nonresponsiveness, and growing metacognitive awareness that he was triggered in the session. He becomes agitated again, this time when describing once having been left alone most of the night as a young child, and the extreme worry he experienced until his parents eventually returned, in an intoxicated state. The therapist responds to this activated memory with encouragement, nonintrusive compassion, and support, and, after 20 minutes of processing, suggests a brief relaxation exercise.]

From a reconsolidation perspective, it is likely that Ben's memories of abandonment and parental unavailability, especially if repeatedly accessed and processed, may become modified through association with new experiences of therapist attention, validation, and caring, increased metacognitive awareness, and a period of relaxation within the reconsolidation window. These activities likely will "subtract" some level of distress from the new, soon-to-be reconsolidated memory, meaning that future triggers will activate less neglect-related emotional pain, and thus lessen the need for a DRB. Additional opportunities for *in vivo* processing in the future will likely contribute to further alteration of this schema.

Steps of Processing

Based on the theory and literature reviewed here, the processing component of RA-focused treatment consists of six steps that address both explicit and implicit memories. Adapted from the self-trauma model (e.g., Briere & Scott, 2014) they are *prebriefing, exposure, activation, disparity/new information, counterconditioning/extinction,* and *debriefing/closure.*

Prebriefing

Prebriefing is recommended for any therapeutic exposure procedure, let alone when applied to DRB-involved clients. This is because, at first glance, exposure interventions seem counterintuitive: Why would anyone specifically seek out activities that produce unwanted emotional states—especially as a supposed way to decrease those states in the future? This question may be especially relevant to those who devote considerable time and effort to distress avoidance in the first place. In the absence of a compelling rationale, the client is likely to resist doing something that feels bad, even if the clinician recommends it. For this reason, it is important that the therapist explain the specific rationale for exposure, and its methodology, so that the client can see the potential real-world benefit. In general, discussion of the following points may be helpful, as presented in Briere and Scott (2014):

- Unresolved trauma and attachment memories usually have to be talked about in order to lose their painful qualities. Although the client may have become expert at avoiding upsetting feelings, such avoidance often has the unfortunate side effect of keeping the trauma alive.

- If the client can talk enough about what happened, unwanted feelings associated with the past are likely to decrease in the future, although this cannot be guaranteed.

- At the same time, by its nature, exposure is usually associated with some level of distress. Some (but not all) people who undergo exposure experience a brief increase in flashbacks, nightmares, and feelings between sessions, but this is a normal response to successful activation. Client feedback in this area is important, however, so that the therapist can monitor whether activation is too uncomfortable or too intense.

- The therapist will work to keep the discussion of these memories from overwhelming the client, and, in contrast to PE, the client can stop talking about any given memory anytime it becomes too upsetting. But the more the client can remember, think, feel, and talk about what happened, without significant avoidance, the more likely significant improvement will occur.

Exposure

Exposure refers to the moment when the individual encounters a reminiscent stimulus or memory cue that triggers a memory or schema. It does not include her response to the stimulus, which is described in the next step. Examples of exposure cues include the following:

- Verbal requests for autobiographical information, including questions from others about a past event.
- Speaking, thinking, or writing about some aspect of the past.
- Contact with media, such as television, radio, movies, or websites that contain reminiscent stimuli.
- Reminiscent people, places, situations, or relationships.
- A specific date or anniversary.
- Sensory stimuli, such as smells, sounds, or being touched in certain ways.
- Perceptions of threat, such as sudden movement near one's face or

body, unwanted sexual stimuli, boundary violations, angry faces, or yelling.

In many of these cases, exposure occurs outside of therapy. In fact, the term *triggering* is generally equivalent to *exposure,* except that the former is often seen as unwanted events in the environment, whereas the latter is typically used in the context of therapy. Apropos of this, triggering outside of therapy may also desensitize memories, and probably contributes to "natural" recovery from traumatic events (Briere, 2002a; Foa, Huppert, & Cahil, 2006).

In therapy, exposure can occur in two separate ways:

1. In the verbal, narrative domain, when the therapist asks the client about her history, or when the client spontaneously discloses it.
2. In the nonverbal and relational domain, often in response to aspects of the therapy environment. These include therapist characteristics (e.g., gender, age, race, ascribed social power), the quality of the therapeutic relationship (e.g., accepting vs. judging, caring vs. dismissing), and the extent to which the therapeutic interaction cues early attachment memories (e.g., perceived lapses in attunement, or, alternatively, protective or caring therapist behaviors).

Exposure as just described does not just occur in cognitive-behavioral therapy. It is also present in relational treatment, when aspects of the therapy process trigger attachment memories. It also occurs in more experiential or expressive therapies, when the client is encouraged to paint, draw, or dramatically reenact the past.

Exposure is, to some extent, the first step in what psychodynamic clinicians refer to as *transference,* in that it involves encountering relational stimuli in the session that are similar to aspects of an important early figure, typically a childhood caretaker. However, most of what is considered transference involves *activation,* as described below.

Activation

Activation occurs whenever exposure to reminiscent stimuli results in emotions, sensations, fear structures, or trauma schemas that were initially conditioned to the adverse event. For example, if the clinician is late for a session or suddenly cannot attend at the scheduled time, the client may think or feel what he experienced in early in childhood, for example, abandonment, rejection, or anger. Importantly, these activation responses are almost always triggered implicit—rather than explicit—memories, and are often experienced in the context of source attribution errors. For example, in the case of therapist lateness activating an abandonment schema, the client may not think "My therapist's behavior is triggering early memories of parental neglect," but rather, "My therapist is dismissive of my needs because he is uncaring and I am unworthy." Although, as noted, this response is sometimes described as transferential, an RA perspective considers it an example of implicit activation. This view is in contrast to a classically psychoanalytic perspective on transference, in which the client is thought to unconsciously "redirect" (Freud, 1912/1958) conflict-related emotions and thoughts from a childhood figure to the therapist.

As noted elsewhere, activated emotions and thoughts can become triggers for additional memories and therefore loop back to the exposure component of treatment. Such trigger chaining means that a given client may experience both the activation of a previously triggered emotion or thought and exposure to a new memory, the latter of which may then activate new emotional distress. The possibility of simultaneously activated emotional states and trigger-chained new memories means that the clinician cannot assume that emotional processing will proceed in a linear fashion. It also reinforces the value of attending to therapeutic window dynamics early in the process, and the importance of the therapist's continuing, moment-by-moment attunement to the client's shifting internal experience.

Trigger chaining aside for the moment, the RA perspective suggests that exposure, alone, generally does not have positive therapeutic effects. Instead, to be helpful, it must activate implicit memories associated with the trauma or attachment breach/failure. This is sometimes observed in clients who are willing to talk about past traumas, but who dissociate, intellectualize, or distract themselves to such an extent that they do not appear to be activated, and do not gain much from the process. They have, of course, been triggered at some level, or they would not need to avoid. However, such avoidance may sufficiently reduce activated distress that meaningful emotional processing cannot occur. In a similar vein, the client who comes to sessions intoxicated may undergo exposure, but the anesthetizing effects of alcohol or drugs may block sufficient activation.

Disparity/New Information

Significantly, even exposure and activation are usually insufficient for trauma/attachment processing. There must also be *disparity*, or lack of agreement between the activated state and what is actually happening in the session (Briere & Scott, 2014). In the absence of disparity, for example, the client might feel that the therapist is rejecting her, and have this impression reinforced by, in fact, the therapist's rejecting behavior. Therapeutic disparity is a form of expectancy violation (Craske et al., 2014):

The client expects rejection, but that expectation is not supported in the session.

In this way, disparity provides the ingredients for extinction: As the client repeatedly feels or expects rejection, in the absence of it actually occurring, new learning begins to compete with childhood memories. Instead of "My therapist's silence means she doesn't care about me," for example, the client may learn by direct experience that therapeutic silence does not presage rejection or abandonment. In fact, as discussed in the next step, it may reflect active listening, empathy, and attunement. Similarly, the client may discover in a safe therapeutic relationship that vulnerability does not have to lead to injury, connection is not always a precursor to loss, and struggling with entitlement and self-affirmation does not necessarily result in punishment from not knowing one's place.

Simply stated, the exposure–activation–disparity sequence means that treatment of painful trauma/attachment memories best occurs when the client feels triggered distress but there is little in the current environment about which to be upset. This can take place in personal relationships, but it is more efficiently supported in therapy, where safety is ideally assured, and exposure and activation are titrated so that they do not overwhelm. Notably, if activation is too great, or the therapist is overwhelmed or insufficiently supportive, disparity will not be present. Instead of feeling moderate levels of distress in the absence of reinforcement, the client may experience overwhelmingly negative emotional and cognitive states, which, given their threatening qualities, do not contribute to extinction of the trigger–memory connection. In fact, when memories are allowed to repeatedly overwhelm, the client may become resensitized, not desensitized.

It is in this context that the therapeutic window, described earlier, becomes relevant. The *therapeutic window* refers to the psychological space between insufficient and excessive exposure and activation. Mid-window interventions are neither so nondemanding that they provide inadequate exposure and processing nor so evocative or powerful that they overwhelm. Overshooting the therapeutic window occurs when activation is too intense or involves premature exposure to aspects of memory that requires additional processing before they can be addressed in their entirety.

The therapeutic window also can be exceeded when the client or therapist brings up too much material in too short a time. Exposure that moves too fast may overshoot the window, because it does not allow the client to adequately process previously activated material before new, additionally stressful memories appear. When therapy consistently overshoots the window, the survivor must engage in avoidance behaviors in order to keep from being overwhelmed, or even retraumatized, by the therapy process. And, if such activation is not resolved by the end of the session, the client may have to resort to DRBs to regain equilibrium.

Ultimately, the safety component of RA-focused therapy does not just refer to safety from immediate danger, or from harsh or disengaged behavior by the therapist. It also involves titrated processing, whereby the therapist facilitates access to memories, but, at the same time, works to keep these recollections within the therapeutic window, so that they are not overly intense or prolonged. In some cases, especially when exposure is substantial, this involves interspersing interventions that increase resilience to activation, as described in Chapter 7, including grounding, relaxation, self-soothing, positive self-talk, and, when appropriate, movement to less upsetting memories or issues.

It should be noted that concerns about overwhelming the client during therapeutic exposure do not mean that some form of exposure at some point in therapy is contraindicated, even for clients with limited emotional regulation. Although this argument is sometimes made, research suggests that carefully performed therapeutic exposure generally does not lead to retraumatization or especially exacerbated emotional states (e.g., Foa, Zoellner, Feeny, Hembree, & Alvarez-Conrad, 2002). Instead, the issue is usually whether the therapeutic window has been exceeded, such that existing emotional regulation capacities are overwhelmed.

Interspersal and Counterconditioning

Although repeated activation with disparity may be sufficient for extinction of certain memories, especially less relational ones, other memories may require therapeutic counterconditioning. The positive feelings the client experiences in the context of the therapeutic relationship, and the positive valence of interspersal activities like relaxation or mindfulness, may be a countervailing force when the client is accessing painful memories or is triggered by reminiscent aspect of the therapy. Thus, for example, a client who is discussing sexual abuse by a parent may have the experience of two, simultaneous processes: triggered memories of sexual violation, yet feelings of safety, acceptance, and compassion from another attachment figure. Or, even more paradoxically, the client may have triggered expectations or perceptions of therapist dismissiveness, yet, at the same time, experience "real-time" boundary-aware caring and attunement from him. When these activated memories are reconsolidated, they will likely be encoded with less distress and more positive associations.

Neurobiology

The attachment-based components of therapeutic counterconditioning exceed the mere appreciation that one is being treated well. In fact, there are inborn reinforcements for sustained and intimate human connection, probably arising from the evolutionary need for the child to maximize attachment with caretakers, and vice versa, in a potentially dangerous environment (Bowlby, 1973). Apropos of this, it appears that attachment bonds are rewarded neurobiologically, primarily in terms of triggered oxytocin and related (e.g., dopaminergic) neurochemical release (Strathearn, 2012). Oxytocin, in turn, increases well-being, openness, and willingness to trust others, and down-regulates stress responses and anxiety (e.g., Kirsch et al., 2005; Kosfeld, Heinrichs, Zak, Fischbacher, & Fehr, 2005). Thus, to the extent that therapy activates attachment neurochemistry, the client is likely to experience the classic counterconditioning scenario: exposure to painful memories in the presence of relative well-being and reduced anxiety. This neurobiology suggests the value of therapeutic connections that are secure, caring, and of sufficient duration for some level of attachment biology to take place.

Counterconditioning may also take place when the client cries while remembering painful things. A small literature suggests that "having a good cry" can be cathartic and self-soothing, may trigger oxytocin release, and, especially when done in the presence of a supportive other, decrease stress and improve mood (e.g., Gračanin, Bylsma, & Vingerhoets, 2014; Hendriks, Rottenberg, & Vingerhoets, 2007). In this context, crying while remembering in a supportive environment may countercondition memories with positive feelings associated with emotional release and attachment neurochemistry.

Debriefing/Closure

Research as far back as the 1920s and 1930s (i.e., Lewin, 1935; Zeigarnik, 1927) indicates that incomplete mental processes tend to remain active until they are completed. This *Zeigarnik effect* predicts that memory activation without closure can result in "task-specific tension," which, in turn, keeps the memory active. Fifty years later, Rachman (1980) similarly suggested that unresolved memories tend to intrude into awareness until they are emotionally processed.

These theories are highly relevant to trauma/attachment processing. Because many DRB-involved clients struggle with strongly activated memories, it is important that there be a degree of closure following any given processing episode. This generally occurs when exposure and activation have had a chance to respond to disparity and the therapeutic relationship, and any meaning that can be ascribed to what was discussed has been highlighted. This typically involves a slow shift away from emotionally laden recollections to the "here and now," as the session reaches its predictable end. In many cases, this will include debriefing about what the client experienced during the session, so that any unresolved details or emotional states can be addressed, and a coherent narrative (Amir, Stafford, Freshman, & Foa, 1998) of the session can be formed.

The goal of such actions is for the client to leave the session in at least no more arousal than when he entered it, and, ideally, with a greater sense of meaning or understanding. In some cases, this may be reinforced by the therapist engaging in a reliable "ending ritual" (Linehan, 1993), such as walking the client to the door, noting the next appointment time, and offering a handshake (if appropriate) that signals a positive conclusion to the session.

A Note on EMDR

EMDR (Shapiro, 1998, 2017), a widely used approach to treatment of psychological trauma, has been shown to be generally as effective as classic therapeutic exposure in reducing the symptoms of PTSD (e.g., Lee & Cuijpers, 2013; Seidler & Wagner, 2006). Unfortunately, beyond several case reports (e.g., Korn & Leeds, 2002), there is little research demonstrating the effectiveness of EMDR in treating symptoms or problems beyond posttraumatic stress—particularly complex posttraumatic outcomes such as DRBs, emotional dysregulation, attachment disturbance, or negative relational schemas. As well, van der Kolk and colleagues (2007) report that at 6-month follow-up, EMDR was considerably more effective in eliminating PTSD symptoms among those with adult-onset traumas than among those who had experienced childhood trauma. These results suggest that EMDR may be more efficacious for "simple" adult-onset adversities than for childhood trauma, which tends to involve more symptom complexity and comorbidity over time.

Nevertheless, EMDR has many qualities that are similar to an RA perspective, including processing chained memories; attention to cognitive distortions such as shame or guilt; specific attention to early stabilization; and alternation between desensitization and access to internal resources, which likely serves therapeutic window-like functions. Furthermore, although EMDR tends to focus on explicit trauma memories, some writers, not without controversy, suggest that it can be adapted to address implicit, attachment-level memories as well (e.g., Parnell, 2013).

Because most EMDR activities occur internally, with limited verbal interactions with the therapist, the clinician has relatively little control over what the client is processing at any given moment in time and whether, in fact, trigger chaining is occurring. Although this internal focus provides fewer opportunities for relational processing, many therapists nevertheless find EMDR to be most effective in the context of a positive therapeutic relationship, where the clinician can (1) use "cognitive interweaves" (Shapiro, 2017) to highlight maladaptive schemas and encourage self-compassion, and (2) redirect the client to stabilization activities when necessary.

It is likely that EMDR can be an elective component of DRB-focused therapy, perhaps especially when processing of circumscribed ("hot spot") memories is indicated (Briere & Scott, 2014). Importantly, this approach may be most helpful for DRB-involved clients when it is used as an adjunct to RA-based treatment, and embedded within a relational treatment context that includes attention to emotional regulation, attachment, and titrated processing (Korn, 2009).[1]

Clinical Guidelines for Trauma/ Attachment Processing

Although specific treatment planning and implementation are reviewed in Chapter 9, presented below are some clinical implications of memory processing as they relate to those who engage in DRBs or other avoidance behaviors. These principles apply most directly to DRB-involved clients who suffer from a major imbalance between distressing memories and emotional regulation capacities. In less severe instances, some of these suggestions may be more relevant than others.

Safety, Stability, and the Therapeutic Relationship

Before exposure activities are begun in earnest, it is recommended that a good therapeutic alliance and relationship be present, and that the client be sufficiently stable—both environmentally and emotionally—that he can tolerate some level of memory activation. This includes working to keep the client physically safe, providing necessary psychoeducation, and teaching emotional regulation and trigger management skills.

Intensity Control

Early trauma processing should be less intense than later in therapy, and should occur with careful attention to the therapeutic window. The clinical advice "when in doubt, slow down" is especially relevant to work with DRB-involved clients and others with emotional regulation difficulties. It is generally better to undershoot the therapeutic window (i.e., provide less exposure than the client can actually handle) than to overshoot it, because overwhelming exposure/activation experiences can potentially retraumatize, lead to avoidance responses that decrease therapy effectiveness and motivate dropout, and remove the safety/disparity component of extinction learning.

---

[1]The author is indebted to Gill Moreton, who consulted with him on the relative benefits of EMDR for complex trauma presentations.

The relative equilibrium between the client's existing emotional regulation capacity and the amount of memory-related distress she is experiencing (i.e., her activation–regulation balance) can be informally estimated with the ERAS, presented in Appendix 6.

Prebrief and Debrief

Memory processing can be helpful in reducing DRBs over time but can produce distress in the immediate term. Although attention to the therapeutic window decreases the likelihood that memory activation will overwhelm, it is important that the rationale for exposure be explained in detail to the client, and his agreement obtained, before any major trauma processing is initiated. Similarly, after significant exposure and activation has occurred, the client should be debriefed about her experiences and current level of distress, so that further deescalation of triggered states can be provided, if necessary, and closure can be established.

Avoid Overly Extended Exposure

Except in cases in which a client has relatively strong emotional regulation capacities, it is recommended that any given exposure or activation experience be titrated to emotional regulation capacity and, at least initially, not extend beyond 10–20 minutes for DRB-involved clients. Habituation has not been found to be necessary for trauma processing, and modern exposure studies suggest that exposure beyond 30 minutes per session does not confer additional benefits for the average client, let alone those heavily involved in avoidance behaviors such as DRBs or substance use. As noted earlier, decisions about the length and intensity of a given exposure period should ultimately rest with the client, so that she feels in control of the process, potentially is less frightened by it, and is more able to keep activated material from becoming overwhelming. On the other hand, once DRB-involved clients demonstrate (or have developed) the capacity to tolerate 10–20 minutes of exposure, they can experiment with longer exposure periods, if appropriate. These more extended exposure periods should only occur, however, to the extent that the therapeutic window is not exceeded and the client is not overwhelmed.

Intersperse Exposure with Nonexposure Activities

In contrast to PE, reconsolidation and inhibitory learning theories suggests that exposure/activation may be most effective when alternated with periods of visible relational support, relaxation, breath exercises, brief mindfulness activities, or other nonstressful or soothing experiences that reduce stress or anxiety. These interexposure periods also may be good opportunities to gently discuss cognitive distortions and intrusive negative thoughts, in case they can be updated. All these activities take advantage of the reconsolidation process, since they allow modification of activated memory prior to neural reencoding. They may also increase the likelihood that the therapeutic window will not be exceeded, since such intervals allow repeated deescalation.

Be Alert for Implicit Activations

Often, discussion of an explicit trauma memory will trigger one or more implicit memories. When this occurs, the client may respond with strong emotion; thoughts that reflect self-derogation, abandonment, anger, or helplessness; reliving that the therapist cannot detect; and, in some cases, numbing, dissociation, or some other avoidance response. Depending on the situation, the therapist may choose to temporarily discontinue trauma processing and focus on grounding, relaxation exercises, or nontriggering discussion of what has transpired. Triggered implicit memories are not evidence that something has gone wrong, however: It is often possible to work with the client to stay present when such triggering occurs, and to process *in vivo* the memories that underlie the response. This may be facilitated if the client has previously used the TMW (Appendix 5).

Support Multitarget Processing When Relevant

If the client moves from one memory to another, often (but not inevitably) due to trigger chaining, it is recommended that the therapist follow her there, rather than insist on a predetermined memory target. Target switching may occur because

- There are multiple, equally important trauma and/or attachment memories, each of which is available for processing at any given point in treatment.
- One memory has triggered another.
- The previous memory is sufficiently processed, and no longer supersedes other memories.
- The client's growing emotional regulation capacities allow new access to memories that previously were too distressing.
- The client is self-titrating activation responses by moving to a less challenging memory—an adaptive process incorrectly referred to as *resistance* in some treatment models.

In all of these cases, little is lost by following the client's lead—at worst, a specific trauma may not get as much attention as technically possible, at least at that point in time. At best, the client's autonomy is honored, titration is supported, and the complexity of multiple memories of multiple adversities is acknowledged. Because important memories tend to emerge and reemerge in therapy, and longer-term therapy allows the client to revisit any given memory on multiple occasions, there is less need to fully process a given memory at any specific moment in time.

Facilitate Relational Processing of Implicit Memory

The client–therapist relationship can be used to process implicit, attachment-related memories. It is not a placebo or merely a delivery mechanism for support; it is an active ingredient. Moments when the client makes source attribution errors, or misperceives the therapist's intent or behaviors as judgmental, rejecting, or abusive, are opportunities to respond with antithetical caring, validation, and support, as well as gentle clarification. It is important that the therapist not react with defensive or punitive behaviors, since the goal, at one level, is for the client to respond to the therapist based on negative early schemas, then to have these expectations and responses go unreinforced (the therapist does not respond as the original caretaker might have) and, in fact, have them counterconditioned (the therapist responds to an activated schema with warmth, caring, and support).

Do Not Insist on Trauma Processing at Any Given Moment in Therapy

Exposure to, and activation of, trauma- and attachment-related memories is just one part of RA-focused therapy. Especially earlier in treatment, but throughout therapy, other components may be equally or more important, whether involving emotional regulation training, psychoeducation, trigger management, mindfulness exercises, or the support, validation, and relational processing associated with a positive therapeutic relationship. In general, the choice of interventions at any given moment in time is contingent on what appears to be most helpful in light of the client's immediate capacities and challenges.

CHAPTER 9

Treatment Planning and Implementation

BRINGING IT ALL TOGETHER

This chapter brings together the theory and practice of RA-focused therapy, and suggests the staging of interventions as the client progresses through treatment. Given the complexities of each client's situation and functioning (i.e., severity of past trauma, level of attachment security, current symptomatology, current emotional regulation skills, types and severity of DRBs, level of social support, and stressfulness of the psychosocial environment), therapy may be longer or shorter, and some interventions may be more relevant than others. The structure presented here is for a "typical" course of therapy, one that will almost always require adjustment for any given client.

Initial Sessions

The first few sessions of RA-focused treatment ideally involve a combination of three activities: relational connection, early psychoeducation, and assessment. There can be a dynamic tension between these goals, however. Assessment is obviously important, since the complex etiology and inherent riskiness of DRBs demand early information on the client's current psychological state and the specific behaviors she uses to maintain internal homeostasis. Furthermore, carefully timed, gentle questions about the client's past traumas and experiences may be validating and reassuring, to the extent that her pain or struggles have not been taken seriously or understood by others. On the other hand, the risk of dropout may increase when assessment procedures are initiated too quickly and extensively, and without sufficient relational connection, especially when the client requires more immediate attention, support, and reasons for hope.

First Session

For this reason, unless there is a strong reason for immediate assessment and crisis management (e.g., when client is a potential risk to self or others), the first session with DRB-involved clients is often best devoted to activities that increase the client's sense that he is in a safe, supportive environment in which he is "heard" and appreciated. Often, this will involve the stabilization interventions described in Chapter 5, as well as opportunities for the client to discuss current and past difficulties with DRBs, what, in her opinion, underlies these behaviors, and what her life is like at the present moment.

This is usually not the time for the therapist to make interpretations or provide major therapeutic interventions, other than ensuring safety and avoiding excessive memory activation. Instead, the clinician should listen attentively, ask for further details when relevant, and generally respond with compassion and support to the client's story. This is also when the therapist may first express appreciation for the client's bravery, especially in choosing to be vulnerable with a stranger, and engage the hard work of awareness when avoidance no doubt seems the safer option.

When possible, the first session should also include a brief, nontechnical discussion of the RA perspective on DRBs, and a brief overview of how treatment generally unfolds, including the extent of client control over the pace and focus of therapy, and the importance of developing additional emotional regulation skills. The clinician should stress early on that the client is not sick or bad, but rather is doing the best she can given the distress she feels and her lack of ways to internally regulate these states.

Second and Third Sessions

The next two sessions of RA-focused therapy continue the stabilization, relational, and psychoeducational activities of the first session and—assuming there are no major safety issues—also begin the process of formal assessment. Two RA-focused interviews may be administered at this point: the Review of Distress Reduction Behaviors (Rev-DRB) and the Trigger Review (TR), as well as any relevant psychological tests (see Chapter 4). Apropos of the need to provide as much relational "frontloading" as possible in the first few sessions, these measures should be completed in conversational interactions between client and therapist, as opposed to rote, item-by-item administration. If psychological testing is also included, it is suggested that the client either come in before the session to complete these measures, so that therapy time is not taken up by assessment procedures or, if not contraindicated by any standardized testing requirements, take tests home with him, and return them in the next session.

Review of Distress Reduction Behaviors

The Rev-DRB (presented in Appendix 2) is completed by the client, typically early in the session, with the therapist's assistance. It reviews all the DRBs described in this book, without reference to labels or jargon, and asks the client to indicate the first, last, and total number of times each was used, and specifically how many times in the last 6 months, the last week, and the last day it has occurred. The client can read these items to herself, or the therapist can read them out loud, depending on the client's preference. Endorsement of items on the Rev-DRB allows the client and therapist to consider the client's DRB use over the lifespan, as well as to identify what behaviors are of current concern. Some individuals endorse only one DRB on the Rev-DRB, but others report multiple DRBs within the same time frame. When the latter occurs, the client may pick the DRB that is most problematic to work on first, or, alternatively, the easiest to address, or he may choose to address all DRBs at the same time, based on their co-occurrence and functional similarity (see Chapter 10 for additional consideration of multiple DRB presentations).

It is important that the therapist emphasize during completion of the Rev-DRB that the goal is not to inventory the client's failings or pathologies, but rather to more fully understand what the client has had to do to survive triggered trauma- and/or attachment-related memories. As well, it is recommended that there be sufficient time in the session following the Rev-DRB for the client to debrief with the therapist any shame or negative cognitions that may have been triggered by discussing unwanted behavior.

See the Rev-DRB in Figure 9.1, completed by a hypothetical client.

Trigger Review

The TR (presented in Appendix 3) is generally administered after the Rev-DRB, either in the same session or the following one, depending on logistics and the client's emotional state. It begins with a definition of triggering, specifically, "A trigger is something that reminds you of a bad or upsetting thing in your past, and causes you to suddenly feel like you are back when it happened, or to have the emotions or thoughts you had back then. Most people have a few triggers. What are yours?"

Review of Distress Reduction Behaviors (Rev-DRB)

Client name: _Saul X._   Date: _1/12/19_

Behavior	Age first time ever used	Age last time ever used	Number of times in life (estimate)	Used in the last month? Y = yes N = no	Number of times in the last 6 months (estimate)	Number of times in the last week	Number of times in the last 24 hours
Cutting or burning yourself, banging your head, or hurting yourself in some other way, without wanting to commit suicide	9	23	300	(Y) N	20	5	2
Attempting suicide because you were upset about something that happened or because of an argument	17	22	3	Y (N)	0	0	0
Using sex to calm down or to feel better, or because you couldn't stop yourself	15	22	15	(Y) N	3	1	1
Eating more food than you needed, to calm down or to feel better, or because you couldn't stop yourself	16	23	30	(Y) N	4	1	0
Gambling to calm down or to feel better, or because you couldn't stop yourself	never	never	0	Y (N)	0	0	0

(continued)

FIGURE 9.1. Example of a completed Rev-DRB.

Behavior	Age first time ever used	Age last time ever used	Number of times in life (estimate)	Used in the last month? Y = yes N = no	Number of times in the last 6 months (estimate)	Number of times in the last week	Number of times in the last 24 hours
Stealing things to calm down or to feel better, or because you couldn't stop yourself	never	never	0	Y **Ⓝ**	0	0	0
Buying things you didn't really want or need, to calm down or to feel better, or because you couldn't stop yourself	never	never	0	Y **Ⓝ**	0	0	0
Physically fighting or hitting someone because you were upset about something that happened or because of an argument	16	19	10	Y **Ⓝ**	0	0	0
Picking at your skin or scabs, or pulling out your hair to calm down or to feel better, or because you couldn't stop yourself	15	22	10	**Ⓨ** N	1	1	0
Setting fires to calm down or to feel better, or because you couldn't stop yourself	never	never	0	Y **Ⓝ**	0	0	0
Using the Internet to calm down or to feel better, or because you couldn't stop yourself	never	never	0	Y **Ⓝ**	0	0	0
Using pornography to calm down or to feel better, or because you couldn't stop yourself	15	23	200	**Ⓨ** N	15	4	1

FIGURE 9.1. *(continued)*

This introduction is sufficient for some clients, but others may require further discussion of triggers and triggering before they can respond to the TR. As well, as described in Chapter 7, some clients may not yet realize that they have been triggered in the past, due to source attribution errors or the conceptual novelty of triggering per se. For this reason, the clinician may choose to administer the TR at least twice: first in the early sessions, then later in therapy, when the client is more familiar with triggers and their effects.

The TR consists of two sections: The first is a list of the most common triggers reported by trauma survivors, and the second asks about the client's internal responses to the three most problematic of these triggers. Typically, the client's responses to the top three triggers are sufficient to outline his major triggers and responses. If more are required, the last page of the TR can be copied to provide additional ratings. Because clients often discover additional triggers during RA-focused treatment, the last page of ratings also can be used later in therapy to add further triggers and responses.

As is true for the Rev-DRB, the TR is best completed in the context of a discussion between client and therapist, wherein the client explores and describes his triggers and responses, and determines which are most problematic. Not only does it assess the client's trigger process, it also supports and reinforces metacognitive awareness of the reality of triggering, and the client's own specific triggerability. It also can serve as a way for the client to hypothesize a future triggered state when it otherwise might not be clear. For example, if the client is triggered but does not notice or recognize the trigger, previous experiences with the TR might suggest that his sudden, intrusive anxiety, shame, and self-hatred reflect a heretofore unidentified triggered state, which can then be addressed as such.

See the TR in Figure 9.2, completed by a hypothetical client.

Early to Midtreatment

Because many DRB-involved people suffer from impaired or underdeveloped emotional regulation capacity, the early stages of RA-focused treatment tend to focus more on building self-regulation skills than on formal trauma processing. In other cases, however, the client may have sufficient emotional regulation abilities, but the level of triggered activation she experiences is sufficiently intense that it nevertheless overwhelms her internal resources. The client's activation–regulation balance also can be affected by the amount of stress, danger, and nonsupport in her immediate social and physical environment. This variability from client to client, and from one point in time to another, requires the therapist

Trigger Review (TR)

Client name: _Emma R._   Date: _9/2/19_

A trigger is something that reminds you of a bad or upsetting thing in your past, and causes you to suddenly feel like you are back when it happened, or to have the emotions or thoughts you had back then. Most people have a few triggers. What are yours?

Someone crying _____

Feeling abandoned or rejected _X_

Sexual things _X_

Criticism _X_

Someone being very angry _____

Someone who is drunk or high _____

Someone raising their hand near you _____

Someone saying mean or abusive things to you _X_

People wanting to be too close _____

Family get-togethers _____

Seeing violence on TV, at the movies, or on the Internet _____

Being alone with someone _____

People in authority _X_

Competition _____

Being touched _____

Being lied to _X_

Someone flirting with you or making sexual statements _____

Someone acting like they are better than you _X_

Someone who reminds you of your mother _____

Someone who reminds you of your father _____

Being let down by someone _X_

Being yelled at _____

Mean or dirty looks _X_

Being laughed at _____

Being accused of something you didn't do _X_

Being ignored _____

Feeling alone _____

(continued)

FIGURE 9.2. Example of a completed TR.

143

Feeling controlled by someone __X__

Other triggers: _____ _____ _____

Pick up to three of your worst triggers from above, and answer the questions below:

Trigger #1: _Feeling abandoned or rejected_ _____

What do you _feel_ when you are triggered? (Mark all that pertain.)

Fear or anxiety __X__ Anger __X__ Sadness ____ Confusion ____

Shame __X__ Disgust ____ Guilt ____ Embarrassment ____

Sexual excitement ____ Hunger ____ Alone __X__ Emptiness ____

Horror ____ Betrayal __X__ Grief ____ Humiliation ____

Of the feelings you chose, which are the worst two? _Anger_____ _Betrayal_____

What do you _think_ when you are triggered? (Mark all that pertain.)

You need to escape ____ You are helpless ____ Things are hopeless ____

You want to hurt yourself __X__ You want to hurt someone else ____

You hate yourself __X__ You hate someone else ____

You have been abandoned __X__ You are ugly or disgusting ____

Nobody loves you __X__ You are in trouble ____ You are going to die ____

You are a bad person ____ Something bad is about to happen ____

You are in danger ____

Of the thoughts you chose, which are the worst two? _Want to hurt myself_ _I hate myself_

What else happens when you are triggered? (Mark all that pertain.)

A flashback ____ You space out or go away in your mind ____ You get a headache ____

Bodily reactions (like rapid heartbeat, shortness of breath, dizziness) ____

Nausea ____ You have to do something to make the feelings go away __X__

You faint or pass out ____

You notice that your reaction is too strong or doesn't fit the situation __X__

Trigger #2: _Someone saying mean or abusive things to me_ _____

What do you _feel_ when you are triggered? (Mark all that pertain.)

Fear or anxiety __X__ Anger __X__ Sadness ____ Confusion ____

Shame __X__ Disgust ____ Guilt __X__ Embarrassment __X__

Sexual excitement ____ Hunger ____ Alone ____ Emptiness ____

Horror ____ Betrayal ____ Grief ____ Humiliation ____

Of the feelings you chose, which are the worst two? _Shame_____ _Anger_____

(continued)

FIGURE 9.2. *(continued)*

What do you _think_ when you are triggered? (Mark all that pertain.)

You need to escape _____ You are helpless _____ Things are hopeless _____

You want to hurt yourself _____ You want to hurt someone else _____

You hate yourself _____ You hate someone else _X_

You have been abandoned _____ You are ugly or disgusting _____

Nobody loves you _____ You are in trouble _____ You are going to die _____

You are a bad person _X_ Something bad is about to happen _X_

You are in danger _____

Of the thoughts you chose, which are the worst two? _I am a bad person_ _I am in trouble_

What else happens when you are triggered? (Mark all that pertain.)

A flashback _X_ You space out or go away in your mind _X_ You get a headache _____

Bodily reactions (like rapid heartbeat, shortness of breath, dizziness) _____

Nausea _____ You have to do something to make the feelings go away _____

You faint or pass out _____

You notice that your reaction is too strong or doesn't fit the situation _X_

Trigger #3: _Feeling controlled by someone_ _____

What do you _feel_ when you are triggered? (Mark all that pertain.)

Fear or anxiety _____	Anger _X_	Sadness _____	Confusion _____
Shame _____	Disgust _____	Guilt _____	Embarrassment _____
Sexual excitement _____	Hunger _____	Alone _____	Emptiness _____
Horror _____	Betrayal _____	Grief _____	Humiliation _X_

Of the feelings you chose, which are the worst two? _Anger_ _Humiliation_

What do you _think_ when you are triggered? (Mark all that pertain.)

You need to escape _X_ You are helpless _____ Things are hopeless _____

You want to hurt yourself _____ You want to hurt someone else _____

You hate yourself _____ You hate someone else _____

You have been abandoned _____ You are ugly or disgusting _____

Nobody loves you _____ You are in trouble _____ You are going to die _____

You are a bad person _____ Something bad is about to happen _X_

You are in danger _____

Of the thoughts you chose, which are the worst two? _Need to escape_ _Something bad is about to happen_

(continued)

FIGURE 9.2. _(continued)_

What else happens when you are triggered? (Mark all that pertain.)

A flashback _____ You space out or go away in your mind _X_ You get a headache _____

Bodily reactions (like rapid heartbeat, shortness of breath, dizziness) _____

Nausea _____ You have to do something to make the feelings go away _____

You faint or pass out _____

You notice that your reaction is too strong or doesn't fit the situation _X_

Trigger #_____: _No othe triggers_ _____

What do you _feel_ when you are triggered? (Mark all that pertain.)

Fear or anxiety _____	Anger _____	Sadness _____	Confusion _____
Shame _____	Disgust _____	Guilt _____	Embarrassment _____
Sexual excitement _____	Hunger _____	Alone _____	Emptiness _____
Horror _____	Betrayal _____	Grief _____	Humiliation _____

Of the feelings you chose, which are the worst two? _____ _____

What do you _think_ when you are triggered? (Mark all that pertain.)

You need to escape _____   You are helpless _____   Things are hopeless _____

You want to hurt yourself _____   You want to hurt someone else _____

You hate yourself _____   You hate someone else _____

You have been abandoned _____   You are ugly or disgusting _____

Nobody loves you _____   You are in trouble _____   You are going to die _____

You are a bad person _____   Something bad is about to happen _____

You are in danger _____

Of the thoughts you chose, which are the worst two? _____ _____

What else happens when you are triggered? (Mark all that pertain.)

A flashback _____ You space out or go away in your mind _____ You get a headache _____

Bodily reactions (like rapid heartbeat, shortness of breath, dizziness) _____

Nausea _____ You have to do something to make the feelings go away _____

You faint or pass out _____

You notice that your reaction is too strong or doesn't fit the situation _____

FIGURE 9.2. _(continued)_

to regularly determine the client's current emotional regulation capacity and the extent to which the client can be triggered into painful states. This assessment is facilitated by the In-Session Emotional Regulation and Activation Scale (ERAS; see below and in Appendix 6), which is typically completed by the therapist at the end of each session and reviewed at the beginning of the next session.

In-Session Emotional Regulation and Activation Scale

The ERAS reflects the therapist's subjective estimates of the extent to which the client exhibits (1) emotional regulation capacity and (2) memory activation within any given session, each rated on a scale of 1–4.

Emotional regulation is evaluated by five therapist ratings that reflect the client's session-specific:

1. *Down-regulation capacity* (the extent to which the client was able to calm herself down without using avoidance).
2. *Distress tolerance* (the extent to which the client was able to experience unwanted emotions without engaging in within-session DRBs such as yelling, verbal aggression, hitting himself, or throwing things).
3. *Tendency to be overwhelmed by activation* (the extent to which the client was able to experience distress without becoming highly upset or disorganized).
4. *Metacognitive awareness* (the extent to which the client was able to demonstrate metacognitive awareness in the session).
5. *Level of dissociation* (the extent to which the client engaged in dissociation, such as "spacing out," a monotonous voice, or having derealization or depersonalization experiences in the session).

After completing these ratings, the therapist then provides an *overall estimate of emotional regulation this session,* ranging from *low* to *high.* Although this score may be the average of all five ratings, it is intended to summarize the therapist's evaluation of the client's overall emotional dysregulation. As a result, the therapist may endorse a summary score that is not a simple function of the five items, but rather reflects additional perceptions of the client's capacity to regulate distress.

Estimation of *level of activation* is based on five therapist ratings of the client's session-specific:

1. *Triggerability* (the extent to which the client is easily triggered in the session, typically by relational or attachment-related stimuli).
2. *Intensity of triggered activation* (the intensity or magnitude of triggered responses in the session).

3. *Duration of triggered activation* (the duration of triggered responses in the session; e.g., seconds or minutes).
4. *Activated anger* (level of triggered anger in the session).
5. *Level of reliving* (the extent to which triggering results in temporary breaks from current reality, in the form of reliving responses in the session).

Following these ratings, the therapist then assigns an *overall estimate of memory activation this session* score, ranging from *low* to *high*. As with the emotional dysregulation score, this summary may or may not consist of the average of individual activation items.

The relationship between emotional dysregulation and level of activation scores allows the clinician to estimate the client's activation–regulation balance, and thus which interventions may be most useful and least problematic. This estimation is, however, based on the previous session, and therefore should be modified by any information at the beginning of the current session that suggests additional intervening factors. For example, although the ERAS might indicate that, based on the previous session, the client has a reasonably good activation–regulation balance, it may be that between-session circumstances (e.g., a relationship breakup, inadequate sleep, or new victimization experience) tilt the current activation–regulation balance toward overactivation; therefore, stabilizing interventions might be more indicated than previously thought.

See the ERAS in Figure 9.3, completed by a therapist.

Harm Reduction

In instances in which one or more DRBs are creating risk, whether to health, relationships, or social functioning, the harm reduction interventions described in Chapter 5 are best introduced early in treatment, usually before major trauma processing is begun. This may occur at the same time as emotional regulation skills development, but it is a greater priority for treatment when it is relevant. For example, an individual who is self-cutting obviously will gain from emotional regulation interventions, but it may be even more important to help him find ways to reduce the severity of this behavior so that inadvertent life risk or disfigurement is less likely. As described in Chapter 5, short of hospitalization or other extreme interventions, harm reduction interventions include:

- Attempting to delay avoidance behaviors for as long as possible after the onset of a trigger.
- When possible using distraction behaviors in lieu of DRBs or, failing that, replacing dangerous DRBs with less detrimental behaviors.
- Or, if DRBs are impossible to avoid, consciously engaging in the behavior to the least extent possible.

In-Session Emotional Regulation and Activation Scale (ERAS)

Client name: *Mohammed M.*   Date: *2/17/18*

Estimated Level of Emotional Regulation This Session

		1	2	3	4
1.	**Down-regulation capacity in session**	Low	②	3	High
2.	**Distress tolerance in session**	Low	②	3	High
3.	**Tendency to be overwhelmed by activation**	1 High	2	③	4 Low
4.	**Metacognitive awareness in session**	① Low	2	3	4 High
5.	**Level of dissociation in session**	1 High	2	③	4 Low
	Overall estimate of emotional regulation this session	1 Low	②	3	4 High

Estimated Level of Activation This Session

		1	2	3	4
1.	**Triggerability in session**	1 Low	2	③	4 High
2.	**Intensity of triggered activation**	1 Low	2	③	4 High
3.	**Duration of triggered activation**	1 Short	2	③	4 Extended
4.	**Level of activated anger**	1 Low	2	3	④ High
5.	**Level of reliving**	1 Low	②	3	4 High
	Overall estimate of memory activation this session	1 Low	2	③	4 High

Activation–Regulation Balance This Session

1	2	3	4
Overactivated	②	3	Well-regulated

FIGURE 9.3. Example of a completed ERAS.

In the case of potentially harmful self-injury, for example, the client who feels the urge to cut on himself might:

- Try "sitting with" the feeling while intentionally not engaging in self-injury for as long as possible, perhaps using the urge-surfing approach outlined in Chapter 6, so that the feeling lessens in intensity over time and does not have to be acted on.
- If the need to "do something" eventually supersedes delaying and urge surfing, engaging in a distracting behavior, whether it be exercise, walking around the block, going for a run, or calling a friend.
- Or, if self-injurious behavior is absolutely impossible to resist, engaging in reduced-level replacement activities such as snapping a rubber band on one's wrist, holding ice cubes in one's hand, doing push-up beyond one's comfort level, or holding one's breath for as long as one can. (Note: It is recommended that the therapist never suggest even low-level physical self-injury).

As noted in the harm reduction literature, these attenuated behaviors are not what we wish for our clients. Ideally, they will be able to develop enough emotional regulation capacities, and/or sufficiently processes attachment or trauma memories, that no form of pain induction is necessary. But these approaches take time, and the client must be kept as safe as possible in the meantime. This may mean that the client continues to be involved in some lower-level DRBs early in treatment.

Emotional Regulation Skills Development and Trigger Management

Either following or simultaneous with harm reduction, the client whose activation–regulation balance skews toward overwhelming internal experiences should be taught emotional regulation and trigger management skills before significant trauma processing is initiated.

Among the activities that can be taught, per previous chapters, are:

- Proactive resilience, including attending to wellness, healthy eating, sleep, and sufficient exercise
- Grounding
- Self-soothing and positive/metacognitive self-talk
- Seeking out relational resources
- Relaxation and breath training
- Strategic distraction
- Emotional detective work

- Meditation and mindfulness, as well as yoga or *tai chi*
- Urge surfing
- Trigger management approaches described in Chapter 7, including trigger identification, the ReGAIN procedure, and other activities that increase metacognitive awareness of triggered states.

Functions of Distress Reduction Behaviors

Although the previous activities can increase the client's general capacity to regulate triggered emotional states, the F-DRB checklist (presented in Appendix 4) also may be used to target specific DRB-motivating phenomena. As noted earlier, this checklist evaluates the psychological functions of each DRB endorsed by the client. For example, if the client reports compulsive binge eating, he might identify several reasons for this behavior, such as distraction from triggered emotional states, memory blocking, self-soothing, and relief from unwanted dissociation. After identifying these reasons, the client and therapist can then pick emotional regulation or trigger management activities that serve generally equivalent functions or otherwise address these specific needs. The bingeing client, for example, might specifically utilize strategic distraction and grounding exercises to address his need to pull attention away from triggered distress, unwanted memories, and dissociation; self-soothing and self-talk activities as alternatives to using food to calm himself; and ReGAIN and mindfulness training to decrease reactivity to relational stimuli that trigger bingeing episodes.

See the F-DRB checklist in Figure 9.4, completed by a hypothetical client.

Attachment and Trauma Processing

Although major attachment–trauma processing is more prevalent later in treatment with DRB-involved clients, those who have stronger emotional regulation capacities, or less severe attachment/trauma memories, may gain from some degree of emotional processing in earlier sessions. In such cases, the clinician may gain from consulting ERASs from the last several sessions to determine the client's overall activation–regulation balance. In general, the more the activation–regulation balance trends toward regulation, the more emotional processing can occur. Some of this processing gradient happens naturally: Clients with greater activation than regulation tend to use more avoidance within sessions and therefore process less, whereas those more on the regulated end of the continuum may be able to experience more distress without being overwhelmed and are therefore more open to processing.

Functions of Distress Reduction Behaviors (F-DRB)

Client name: _Alexa D._   Date: _9/8/19_

From the following list, pick up to three behaviors that you most want to change.

#1. Cutting or burning yourself, banging your head, or hurting yourself in some other way without wanting to commit suicide _X_

#2. Attempting suicide because you were upset about something that happened or because of an argument ____

#3. Sexual behavior that got you into trouble or created problems for you _X_

#4. Binge eating ____

#5. Gambling that got you into trouble or created problems for you ____

#6. Stealing things that you didn't really need ____

#7. Buying things you didn't really need ____

#8. Physically fighting or hitting someone because you were upset about something that happened ____

#9. Picking at your skin or scabs, or pulling out your hair ____

#10. Setting fires ____

#11. Using the Internet so much that you had problems in relationships, at work, or personally ____

#12. Using pornography so much that you had problems in relationships, at work, or personally _X_

Now, indicate the reasons why you use each one.

Behavior (write the # and a brief description): _1. Cutting myself_

_____

_____

Reasons for behavior

To distract yourself from your problems _X_   To stop feeling numb ____

To let people know how you feel ____   To stop memories ____

To block thoughts ____   To stop upsetting feelings _X_

To stop a flashback ____   To feel good so you couldn't feel bad ____

To feel important ____   To control others ____

To get the anger out _X_   To punish yourself _X_

To feel back in your body ____   To get even with someone ____

So someone would pay attention to you ____   To soothe yourself ____

To feel connection with someone ____   To stop feeling empty ____

(continued)

FIGURE 9.4. Example of a completed F-DRB checklist.

Behavior (write the # and a brief description): 3. *Having sex all the time*
_____
_____

Reasons for behavior

To distract yourself from your problems _X_	To stop feeling numb ____
To let people know how you feel ____	To stop memories ____
To block thoughts ____	To stop upsetting feelings _X_
To stop a flashback ____	To feel good so you couldn't feel bad _X_
To feel important _X_	To control others ____
To get the anger out ____	To punish yourself ____
To feel back in your body ____	To get even with someone ____
So someone would pay attention to you _X_	To soothe yourself ____
To feel connection with someone _X_	To stop feeling empty _X_

Behavior (write the # and a brief description): 12. *Using pornography*
_____
_____

Reasons for behavior

To distract yourself from your problems _X_	To stop feeling numb ____
To let people know how you feel ____	To stop memories ____
To block thoughts ____	To stop upsetting feelings _X_
To stop a flashback ____	To feel good so you couldn't feel bad _X_
To feel important ____	To control others ____
To get the anger out ____	To punish yourself ____
To feel back in your body ____	To get even with someone ____
So someone would pay attention to you ____	To soothe yourself _X_
To feel connection with someone ____	To stop feeling empty ____

FIGURE 9.4. *(continued)*

Processing that occurs earlier in treatment must especially occur within the therapeutic window, where, as described in Chapter 8, activation is titrated to match existing emotional regulation capacity. In some cases, this means that exposure activities are constrained to shorter periods of time and are less intense in nature. This is true not only when processing discrete, verbal memories but also when implicit relational memories require attention. Titrated relational processing in this context typically means, for example, that the therapist is especially nonconfrontational with those who were chronically criticized as children, especially present and attuned for those with abandonment issues, and especially attentive to even minor boundary issues in work with those who were exploited or sexually victimized. In each case, the amount of potential relational activation is limited to the extent possible, so that triggering is less intense and therefore less overwhelming.

Mid- to Late Treatment

As treatment progresses, and the client's activation–regulation balance begins to shift away from overwhelming states, the focus of therapy shifts as well. When the client develops greater emotional regulation capacities, less stabilization is required, as well as less emotional regulation training and trigger management. In contrast, attachment and trauma processing may now be more possible, because increased emotional resources means that greater therapeutic exposure to distressing memories can occur

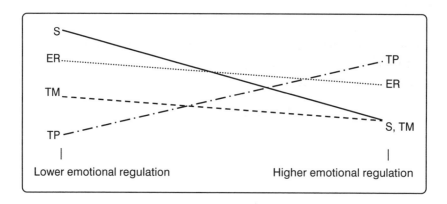

FIGURE 9.5. Suggested level of component use based on overall emotional regulation capacity. S, stabilize/support; ER, Emotional regulation training; TM, trigger management; TP, titrated processing.

without overwhelming the client and triggering further avoidance. However, even later in treatment, the DRB-involved client may easily require continued attention to safety, emotional regulation, and trigger management, albeit typically at reduced levels. See Figure 9.5 for a graphical representation of how treatment components may vary as a function of growing emotional regulation capacity.

"Deeper" Memory Processing

Although, as noted, some level of attachment–trauma processing can occur earlier in treatment, work in this area becomes more central as the client's activation–regulation balance improves and she is able to tolerate more direct, albeit still titrated, exposure to implicit and explicit memories. Even though the intensity of therapeutic exposure is increased, processing nevertheless (1) must occur within the therapeutic window; (2) may shift between multiple client-guided memory targets; (3) should be interspersed with less distressing, nonexposure therapeutic activities; and (4) must occur in the context of visible therapist caring and support.

An important aspect of later-term attachment–trauma processing is the effect of the client's growing attachment to the therapist and the overall strengthening of the therapeutic relationship. Not only does a strong therapeutic relationship increase the client's investment in psychotherapy, it is likely that the client's deepening emotional connection to the therapist will activate neurochemistry (e.g., oxytocin) that has evolved in humans to reward attachment bonds. As described earlier, the effects of such chemical release include a subjective sense of well-being, a willingness to be emotionally vulnerable, and increased feelings of trust, as well as down-regulated stress and anxiety. These internal experiences, in turn, likely serve as powerful counterconditioners when upsetting memories are (1) activated, (2) altered by the presence of positive states, then (3) reconsolidated in longer-term treatment.

Finally, the neurobiology of attachment may temporarily boost the client's emotional regulation capacity, allowing the therapist to act as an "interactive psychobiological regulator" (Schore, 1994) during the treatment session, thereby permitting greater emotional processing of challenging memories. In this regard, several decades of studies (see reviews by Palumbo et al. [2017] and Kleinbub [2017]) suggest that therapist empathy and rapport may allow the client to neurobiologically synchronize with the emotionally regulated and grounded clinician and downregulate his own sympathetic nervous system activity within the therapy session (e.g., Stratford, Lal, and Meara [2012]).

For these reasons, the mid- to late portions of sustained therapy are often experienced by client and therapist as most productive and sometimes most enjoyable. Therapy often is most intense and efficient once the therapeutic relationship has deepened, the client's activation–regulation balance is optimized, and he is less defended and more open to psychotherapy. At the same time, however, attachment dynamics that are activated by the therapeutic relationship can also trigger implicit memories of attachment breaches or maltreatment. The good news about this process is that the client has the opportunity to process important implicit memories that, without sufficient attachment activation, might not otherwise receive attention. The more challenging aspect is that the client may be prone to new source attribution errors, sometimes presenting as increasingly dependent, demanding, or antagonistic behavior (Briere, 1996). Although this can be momentarily discouraging to client and therapist, it is actually a sign of "deeper" work, and, when met with therapist compassion and support, an opportunity for further disparity, counterconditioning, and resolution.

Triggers-to-Memories Worksheet

Memory processing can be aided by use of the Triggers-to-Memories Worksheet (TMW, presented in Appendix 5), in which the client picks up to 10 triggers that are problematic in her life, then, to the extent possible, connects each trigger to one or more specific memories. The function of the TMW is twofold: It facilitates further metacognitive awareness of the triggering process, and it serves as an exposure tool. In the latter context, asking the client to connect specific triggers to specific memories of abuse or neglect can activate recollections that are then available for attenuation and counterconditioning in the context of therapeutic safety, caring, and support. This process may be amplified, when appropriate, by asking the client to describe the memories in relative detail, while keeping the processing within the therapeutic window. Because this activity may be repeated multiple times in treatment, it is often helpful to administer a new TMW on each occasion.

TMW-based processing may be especially efficient in addressing the underlying bases for specific DRBs. This is because the client is being asked to emotionally process the memories that are most likely to be triggered, which are likely the ones that need the most attention. However, this also means that exposure and activation using the TMW may, on occasion, be relatively intense. For this reason, the TMW is usually used later in treatment, when the client has been able to increase his emotion regulation and stabilization skills.

See the TMW in Figure 9.6, completed by a hypothetical client.

Triggers-to-Memories Worksheet (TMW)

Client name: _Saul X_   Date: _1/12/19_

Place checkmarks next to the 5–10 triggers that make you feel the most upset or that produce the biggest problems for you:

Someone crying _X_

Feeling abandoned or rejected ____

Sexual things _X_

Criticism ____

Someone being very angry _X_

Someone who is drunk or high _X_

Someone raising their hand near you _X_

Someone saying mean or abusive things to you ____

People wanting to be too close ____

Family get-togethers _X_

Seeing violence on TV, at the movies, or on the Internet ____

Being alone with someone ____

People in authority _X_

Competition ____

Being touched ____

Being lied to ____

Someone flirting with you or making sexual statements ____

Someone acting like they are better than you ____

Someone who reminds you of your mother ____

Someone who reminds you of your father _X_

Being let down by someone ____

Being yelled at _X_

Mean or dirty looks ____

Being laughed at ____

Being accused of something you didn't do ____

Being ignored ____

Feeling alone ____

Feeling controlled by someonee ____

Other triggers: _____ _____ _____

(continued)

FIGURE 9.6. Example of a completed TMW.

For each of the triggers you chose, try to connect the trigger to a specific upsetting memory or memories of things that happened to you in the past. This may not be possible for some triggers. Just do the best you can.

Trigger	Memory or memories
Someone crying	My mom being beaten up by my dad. My dad dying from a bad liver. My first girlfriend breaking up with me because I cheated on her.
Someone being angry	My mom being beaten by my dad. My dad beating me. Being bullied at school. My first girlfriend breaking up with me because I cheated on her. My teachers.
Someone who is drunk	My mom being beaten up by my dad when he was drunk. My dad beating me. My dad drinking all the time. My friend driving my car when he was drunk, and we crashed.
Someone raising their hand to me	My dad beating me.
Family get-togethers	My mom being beaten by my dad. My dad beating me. My mom and dad fighting all the time. When my brother pulled a gun on my dad at Christmas.
Someone in authority	My dad being mean to everybody. Teachers always saying I was stupid and making fun of me. Cops in my neighborhood putting everyone down and arresting people for no reason.
Someone reminds me of my father	My mom being beaten by my dad. My dad beating me.
Being yelled at	My dad beating me. Being bullied at school. My mom and dad yelling at each other all the time.
Sexual things	My sexual abuse when I was a kid. My first girlfriend breaking up with me because I cheated on her. When I got syphilis.

FIGURE 9.6. (*continued*)

In Vivo Processing

As described in Chapter 8, *in vivo* processing involves taking advantage of triggering that occurs within a given session, wherein the client is asked to mindfully allow and experience the associated activated state in the specific context of therapist support and encouragement. As noted, this task requires considerable metacognitive awareness and emotional regulation skills; hence, it is usually initiated later in therapy, and, as always, kept within the therapeutic window.

Prelude to Termination

Because many DRB-involved clients have had negative attachment experiences, and are therefore hypervigilant to separation or perceived abandonment, it is recommended that the end of therapy be discussed as a regular topic in the last months of RA-focused treatment. Not only does this give the client time to accommodate to the idea of termination, but it also allows her to process the impending loss, so that it is less likely to emerge later as experiences of abandonment. In this regard, some clients' seemingly excessive and "borderline" reactions to termination reflect not so much a pathological inability to separate from attachment figures as insufficient processing of triggered abandonment schemas. In this sense, termination discussions are a form of therapeutic exposure to early loss or rejection.

The Quarter Rule

Concretely, clinical experience suggests that termination issues first be broached in the latter quarter of therapy sessions, for example, in the last three sessions of what is likely to be a 12-session course of treatment, or the last 3 months of what is expected to be a year of therapy. This may seem unnecessarily long for some clients, especially those whose difficulties are less pronounced. However, early discussions may be brief, perhaps just the therapist noting when treatment might end, and inquiring about the client's responses to that eventuality, with more detailed and extended conversation occurring closer to the end date. This process may also be facilitated by asking the client when she would like to end therapy, rather than just announcing the date.

As the client moves toward termination, it is also important to focus again on her support system and coping strategies, so that the therapist's absence does not leave the client without relational connections or ways of dealing with the almost inevitable, and entirely appropriate, grief process. The client's reactions should be normalized and validated, and treated as understandable responses to the end of a valued relationship. In this context, problem solving around support and coping may be presented as the logical next step in the therapy process, just as one might prepare for any other challenging or sad event.

Also included during this discussion should be some sort of contingency for the possibility of future therapy, for example if DRBs return or intensify, or if other psychological issues or stressors emerge. If the clinician is able and willing to see the client again in the future, this availability should be made clear prior to termination, so the client knows that it is an option. On the other hand, if for some reason this is not the case, this should be explained as well, and referrals provided. In either instance, the idea that one may need more therapy in the future should be normalized, so that the client is less likely to avoid later assistance if it is needed.

Final Sessions

The last one to two sessions of RA-focused therapy usually involve very little trauma or attachment processing, if possible. This is because further memory activation might require more than a session or two to process and resolve, leaving the client less settled upon termination. Instead, the therapeutic conversation typically involves the further development of a coherent narrative regarding the client's experiences in therapy, and his reactions to ending treatment. Assuming termination issues have been sufficiently addressed, this process can allow therapy to end "on a good note," in which debriefing has already occurred, and client and therapist have the opportunity to say good-bye in a grounded, nonavoidant, reality-based way. This does not mean that the client (and therapist) may not be sad about the end of a significant relationship, but rather that attachment activations and source attribution errors are less prevalent, and meaningful closure can occur.

CHAPTER 10

Special Considerations
for Certain Distress Reduction
Behaviors and Patterns

The previous chapters of this book have outlined the general RA approach to DRBs, noting common antecedents and functions across different types of distress avoidance. However, there are differences between DRBs as well, and certain constellations of behaviors and comorbidities that complicate therapeutic intervention. In this chapter, clinical approaches to three major DRBs are examined in greater detail: *self-injury, compulsive sexual behavior,* and *bingeing–purging.* Also discussed are several especially problematic clinical scenarios: the client with multiple DRBs; DRBs that occur in the context of problematic substance use; and especially high-risk DRBs that require additional interventions.

Self-Injurious Behavior

Of all the DRBs, self-injury is one of the most perplexing and challenging for clinicians. It is often hard to discriminate from suicidal behavior, the actual injuries can be upsetting to view, and the dramatic nature of the act may trigger feelings of helplessness, yet responsibility, in the therapist. And, of all the DRBs, it is one of the most likely to be triggered by therapy dynamics.

In some cases, the client may use self-injury as a way to communicate distress or anger to the clinician, or to increase the clinician's level of attention to him. Despite the fact that such responses reflect desperation and great need, the clinician can end up feeling manipulated or punished, and her own issues may be triggered in response. In fact, even though the advice in such situations is to continue to respond with empathy and compassion, these capacities may be difficult to marshal when the therapist is feeling especially impinged upon or even threatened.

This is most difficult for the therapist when an episode of self-injury appears to arise from the psychotherapy session itself, and the client attributes her self-harm to the therapist's behavior. When this occurs, the clinician is likely to feel some degree of responsibility; not only is the therapist apparently not helping the client with serious, potentially hazardous behavior, she is being accused of causing it.

This conundrum, which is the basis for many consultation requests, typically has two components: the client's source attribution errors and the clinician's counteractivation responses. Session-specific self-injury usually reflects the trigger-rich environment of the therapeutic relationship. Although in-session activations allow the client to process archaic relational–attachment schemas, they can also can result in feelings of rejection, abandonment, or parental disengagement, which the client attributes to the therapist. In the face of reduced emotional regulation capacities, the client may then engage in self-injury between sessions, and believe that he is appropriately punishing the clinician's bad behaviors or his own, or, based on the therapist's assumed nonresponsiveness, providing evidence of just how badly the client is suffering and needs attention.

While understandable, these client behaviors may easily trigger therapist feelings of inadequacy or helplessness, and result in urges to respond punitively or, alternatively, with guilty attempts to do whatever it takes for the client to not self-injure again. Such client activation and therapist counteractivation can produce a vicious cycle, in which the client continues to self-injure and the therapist increasingly doubts herself, responds reflexively, and potentially reinforces the client's distress, source attribution confusion, and the need for more self-injury.

The "solution" to such entanglements sounds easy but often is hard to do. First, the client's behavior must be met with understanding and nonpitying compassion, and viewed as an opportunity to explore the antecedents and outcomes of in-session triggering. When this occurs successfully, relational processing can take place: The client expects, based on triggered schema, that the therapist will abandon, ignore, or punish, but instead, the clinician responds with the disparity and counterconditioning described in Chapter 8, allowing the client to update childhood learning. This is most possible if the therapist can nonjudgmentally detect his own triggered activations in the context of source attribution awareness and self-compassion. Ultimately, anyone would be upset and triggered if someone he cared about, or was responsible for, was engaged in self-injurious behavior, especially if it was attributed to him. The key is not to blame oneself for blaming oneself or for feeling helpless or even angry;

instead, the clinicians job is, in some sense, to do trigger management on himself, so that activated schemas and memories do not translate into unhelpful behavior.

Several principles are especially relevant to the treatment of self-injury whether it is related to therapy dynamics or otherwise:

• *Do not take self-injurious behavior personally.* The clinician is almost never the actual cause of a client's self-harm, although she may be a trigger, and the client may blame the therapist for its occurrence. As with other DRBs, it is also important to remember the RA perspective that self-injury is not the client's "fault" either. It is, instead, a drastic behavior, typically only chosen in desperation, in the seeming absence of other options. This may not always be apparent, since the client may feel some level of justification, efficacy, or empowerment through such behavior. But self-injury does not solve the underlying problem, so the desperation returns, or even increases.

• *Self-injurious behavior is usually a triggered response to an acute relational stressor.* It rarely occurs in response to steady-state dysphoria alone. As a result, any intervention that either helps the client to "catch" triggering before it goes any further or interrupts the transition from trigger to response is likely to be helpful. As described in previous chapters, interventions for self-injury include trigger identification and metacognitive awareness; delaying DRBs; "urge surfing"; relaxation and mindfulness exercises; self-soothing; opposite actions; ReGAINing; strategic distractions such as exercise, nonbinge eating, reading, writing or painting, dancing, or walking around the block; or accessing resources, such as calling a crisis line, phoning a friend, or cuddling a companion animal.

Importantly, these behaviors should be framed as problem-solving approaches to a concrete problem, self-endangerment, rather than as responses to a communication, control, punishment, or attention-focusing aspect of the therapeutic relationship. The clinician does not shame, blame, or pathologize the client for any interpersonal motives that he might have for self-injury, but instead responds in a compassionate, calm manner that emphasizes the importance of the client's well-being and safety. Similarly, when possible, the therapist does not focus more attention on the client when he has self-injured, but instead is *generally* attentive and caring, so that sudden increased attention to self-injury does not inadvertently reinforce self-injury. Given the sometimes complex relational aspects of this DRB, clinical consultation or supervision is often helpful, regardless of the clinician's level of ability, training, or experience.

• *Always consider the possibility of major suicidality or severe self-harm.* Although self-injurious behavior is typically an attempt to survive activated distress, and thus is somewhat antisuicidal, it is not uncommon for suicidal thoughts and behaviors to co-occur with urges to self-injure (see Chapter 2). Even if death is not likely, self-injury still can be disfiguring. In worrisome cases, for example when there is a risk of serious harm or significant mutilation, the clinician should consider psychiatric evaluation for medication or hospitalization. Although hospitalization is not a long-term solution, it is better to be safe than sorry when life threat, disability, or disfigurement is a real possibility.

• *Use harm reduction sparingly.* Although substitute behaviors (e.g., holding ice cubes or doing more push-ups than comfortable) are recommended by many, and are preferable to more extreme forms of self-harm, these behaviors do not teach distress tolerance, address attachment issues, or help to process memories. Instead, they support pain induction as a way to deal with painful experience, and, in instances in which the goal of self-injurious behavior is self-punishment, may reinforce the validity of self-directed anger or shame.

As a result, the client and therapist may have to walk a tightrope: What is the safest thing the client can do without replicating the problem and reinforcing maladaptive solutions to overwhelming distress? When possible, distraction activities are much preferable to replacement ones. Unfortunately, in some instances, especially earlier in therapy, only harm reduction may suffice, from the client's perspective. For an interesting discussion of this issue from the perspective of someone struggling with self-injurious behavior, see *www.talkspace.com/blog/2017/06/time-retire-self-harm-alternatives.*

Compulsive Sexual Behavior

Many of those engaged in compulsive sexual behavior were sexually abused or insecurely attached early in life, and may be confused from an early age about sexuality, intimacy, love, and relationships, let alone their own worth and entitlement to well-being. Although involvement in compulsive behaviors certainly does not improve things in these areas, some people quickly discover that sexual activity, arousal, and momentary intense connection can soothe, distract from, or temporarily neutralize painful internal states, as well as fill perceived emptiness, confer "specialness," reduce isolation, seemingly increase power over others, and address unmet love or attachment needs. In fact, sex is considered a "primary reinforcer" in psychology (Skinner, 1953), due to its power to motivate behavior. For some individuals, compulsive sex reinforces avoidance learning: If one is sufficiently aroused, dysphoria and other negative states are removed from consciousness, albeit only temporarily.

Some clinicians (e.g., Briggie & Briggie, 2015) and popular press books (e.g., Silverman, 2008) suggest yet another reason for compulsive sexual behavior: Attachment deprivation and childhood experiences of sexual abuse may lead to a confusion between sex and love. In the popular lexicon, some compulsively sexual people appear to be looking for love in all the wrong places. Unlike most other DRBs, compulsive sexual behavior is not only a powerful way to reduce painful internal states but it also serves as a way for people who did not receive sufficient attachment-level caring and connection in childhood to access what they believe to be a proxy for love. Yet such behavior rarely recruits love; it tends to be anonymous, secret, rushed, shameful, and focused on physical sensation. This is bad news–good news for the insecurely attached individual: On the one hand, brief and superficial connections rarely provide the hoped-for intimacy and love; on the other hand, there is a reduced chance of triggered abandonment schema. The investment is low, so the losses are minimized.

The specifics of compulsive sexual behavior have several implications for treatment:

• Because it involves, on one level, momentarily intimate connections with others, it is highly reinforcing for those who suffer from attachment-related hunger for nurturance and love but also fear vulnerability, abandonment, or rejection. Thus, although compulsively sexual clients will be helped by learning emotional regulation skills, they also are likely to require more attention to attachment issues.

Among other things, the therapeutic relationship becomes especially important. Within the context of a safe environment, the client can process implicit attachment schemas and, in many cases, memories of sexual abuse, as well as learn how to engage in closeness without defaulting to sexualized behaviors. For some people, the risk of sexualizing the treatment relationship is obviously greater when the therapist is of the gender/orientation/identity the client finds most attractive. However, some highly sexualized clients may become attracted to the therapist irrespective of preferred physical or sexual characteristics (Briere, 1996).

The possibility of sexualization requires that the therapist strongly reinforce boundaries, and, through studied noninvolvement (Briere, 1996), nonjudgmentally deflect sexualized responses to relatedness in treatment. Whether called *erotic transference* (e.g., Ladson & Welton, 2007) or, from the RA perspective, previously reinforced associations and coping responses, sexual thoughts and feelings about the therapist are not unusual and should not be shamed or stigmatized. Instead, they should be encouraged to extinguish over time, as the client's sexualized behaviors go unreinforced, and are discussed within the context of metacognitive awareness and a greater understanding of his need for actual love and connection, rather than (only) sex.

- More than some other DRBs, compulsive sexual behavior almost always carries with it shame, unacceptability, and some form of self- and other-perceived "bad"ness. As a result, the clinician must especially strive to avoid inadvertently shaming the client and be quick to contextualize compulsive sexual behavior as the logical result of history and the client's need to survive overwhelming negative states. This can be difficult. Sometimes, when the client describes the desperate and seemingly sordid nature of his "hookups," and the amount of shame he feels in response, the unprepared therapist may feel uncomfortable, overwhelmed, and sometimes even repelled or, alternatively, titillated. It is important that the clinician see such reactions as potentially triggered phenomena from her own history, and as the results of the very socialization process that leads the client to feel so much shame. An important aspect of treating compulsive sexual behavior is normalization: not of the risks and suffering involved in seemingly indiscriminate sexual acts, but of the client's attempts to cope with, and reduce, triggered memories of abuse or attachment disturbance. In this vein, although some will disagree, it is recommended that the clinician avoid the terms *promiscuous* or *sex addict* when speaking of compulsive sexual behavior. The latter label, for example, contains two potentially shameful words and may not be especially accurate in the first place.

- Compulsive sexual behaviors are especially dangerous, because they place the individual in unsafe contexts when she is most vulnerable. As noted earlier, frequent, less-discriminant sexual behavior is associated with elevated rates of sexual and physical assaults, and substantially increases the likelihood of life-threatening disease. These dangers can impact the therapeutic relationship, since the presence of life risk increases the need for the clinician to be straightforward about the dangers involved, to give unambiguous advice, and to ensure the client's safety. At the same time, RA-focused treatment is not generally authoritarian or in favor of "top down" interventions in which the therapist informs the client about what is right and what is wrong. It is important that the clinician not lecture or castigate, yet also be clear about the risks involved. This also potentially includes providing information on safer sex practices and safety plans (Briere, 2004; Briere & Jordan, 2004), as well as medical referrals when conditions require it.

- Finally, because compulsive sexual behavior is often associated with insufficient love and nurturance early in life, and subsequent sexual exploitation in childhood, treatment should help the client to increase self-focused capacities. Both sexual abuse and inadequate parental caretaking tend to teach the developing child that his well-being is contingent on pleasing, or accommodating to others, so that her own needs can be met. This false information can be countered in treatment by therapist behaviors that focus on the client's needs, not the clinician's, and that demonstrate that the client does not need to please the therapist in order to receive caring or connection. At a more concrete level, the client may especially need help in developing self-soothing skills, since these are often underdeveloped among those with insecure attachment (Mikulincer & Shaver, 2016).

Bingeing and Purging

Many aspects of binge eating and purging (with or without anorexia) are well explained by the RA model, including the role of attachment difficulties, childhood abuse and neglect, triggering, and inadequate emotional regulation. However, binge eating–purging includes other symptoms and problems as well, including low self-esteem, depression, body dissatisfaction, mental rigidity, and food-related preoccupations (Mayo Clinic; *www. mayoclinic.org/diseases-conditions/bulimia/symptoms-causes/syc-20353615*). These additional issues complicate treatment and often require specific cognitive-behavioral interventions. For this reason, severe cases of BN, BED, and binge-purge anorexia, are best seen by an eating disorder specialist, especially if there are medical risks present.

When bingeing or purging is neither severe nor life threatening, however, the approach described in this book may be sufficient. In any event, an RA approach is not inconsistent with current CBTs (including DBT) for binge–purge behaviors (e.g., Murphy, Straebler, Cooper, & Fairburn, 2010; Safer, Telch, & Chen, 2009), and may be integrated into such protocols as needed. Presented below are several principles of an integrated RA–CBT approach to binge–purge behaviors.

In most treatments for binge eating–purging, the first step is to normalize the client's eating patterns and to address any physical or psychological impacts of disordered eating. This is, essentially, the stabilization phase described in Chapter 5; if the client cannot alter her eating patterns, and the behaviors involved are severe, she is at continued risk of the medical complications (including life risk), also described in Chapter 5. As well, because bingeing and purging can be accompanied by depression, anxiety, suicidality, and/or substance use (O'Brian & Vincent, 2003), interventions should address any comorbidities early on in therapy, before they can complicate treatment or contribute to negative outcomes. This may include, when indicated, the careful use of antidepressants or other psychiatric medication (Gorla & Mathews, 2005). Finally, suicidality is not uncommon among binge eaters or purgers (Koutek, Kocourkova, & Dudova, 2016); thus, continuing lethality assessments may be warranted. In the relatively small number of instances when stabilization cannot be done on an outpatient basis (i.e., when there are critical medical effects of purging, or the client is a danger to himself), referral for short-term hospitalization may be indicated (American Psychiatric Association, 2006).

Following stabilization, the emotional regulation skills development component of RA-focused treatment can be added, including relaxation, trigger management, and use of the ReGAIN procedure. Mindfulness training, DBT, and ACT may be especially helpful for bingeing–purging, to the extent that they increase metacognitive awareness, self-acceptance (vs. low self-esteem and body dissatisfaction) and mindful eating (Masuda & Hill, 2013; Wanden-Berghe, Sanz-Valero, & Wanden-Berghe, 2011).

Importantly, triggering is a significant aspect of binge eating and purging (Lyubomirsky, Casper, & Sousa, 2001). Relational stimuli (e.g., conflict, loss, rejection, abuse reminders) can activate early attachment and abuse memories, leading to a need to binge or to purge as a way to reduce distress through self-soothing, distraction, and filling perceived emptiness. Notably, this type of triggering is not equivalent to what are called *food triggers* in eating disorder treatment, which refer to certain foods, often high in sugars or other carbohydrates, that trigger craving for greater and greater amounts of food. Whereas clients are counseled to avoid food triggers, trigger management involves identifying and directly engaging triggered states, as described in Chapter 7. Trigger management for binge–purge behavior includes:

- Recognizing relational stimuli in the current environment (e.g., rejection) that trigger distressing memories, thoughts, self-perceptions, and emotions, and tend to lead to bingeing or purging.
- Developing metacognitive awareness of triggered states, including body dysmorphia, negative self-appraisals, ruminations, self-disgust, and intrusive urges to eat or purge.
- "Surfing" these urges rather than suppressing them or acting on them.
- Learning how to intervene in triggered states before they can overwhelm and motivate bingeing or purging.

This phase of treatment typically also involves psychoeducation and nutritional counseling regarding the dynamics of bingeing and purging, and RA model principles as they relate to this eating pattern. This includes reinforcing the meal planning skills first introduced during stabilization, including eating regular, portion-controlled meals and snacks, and avoiding trigger foods.

The memory processing phase of RA-focused approaches to DRBs may constitute the next stage of treatment, although there is relatively little discussion of emotional processing in existing binge–purge treatment models. Typically, this involves both titrated exposure to childhood memories of maltreatment and/or neglect and more relational and *in vivo* processing of implicit attachment memories, as described in Chapter 8. Because those who binge and/or purge often struggle with emotional dysregulation and sudden intrusions of self-hatred or self-disgust, therapeutic window dynamics should be especially monitored and controlled during emotional processing.

Like compulsive sexual behaviors, bingeing and purging behaviors are especially associated with shame, which may then support further bingeing and purging. For this reason, it is critical that the behavior of clients who binge and purge be normalized and depathologized throughout treatment, using the RA perspective. Ideally, this involves the client's clear understanding that her behavior is neither good nor bad, but is entirely understandable based on factors that were not under her control, but that now may be addressed.

Multiple DRBs

Kazimir is a 20-year-old man who carries diagnoses of BPD, intermittent explosive disorder, and alcohol use disorder at his local mental health center. His chart documents a long history of self-injury, problematic sexual behavior, and suicide attempts, as well as periods of excessive drinking. Kazimir was adopted from an out-of-country orphanage at age 4 by a supportive and caring couple, with whom he lived until age 18. During that time, he saw many therapists for what was diagnosed as a reactive attachment disorder. His parents report that Kazimir becomes highly distressed upon any perceived evidence of rejection, dismissiveness, disattunement, or abandonment, after which he typically engages in aggression or self-injury.

As noted in the early chapters of this book, it is not uncommon for someone who engages in one DRB to also engage in others. There are at least two reasons for this. Because all DRBs serve the same general purpose of distress avoidance, it is not surprising that those with overwhelming internal states might use several of them. As well, research on *complex trauma exposure* (i.e., the experience of having been victimized in multiple ways in childhood and later in life, as is often the case for DRB-involved people), is associated with having a range of symptoms or problem behaviors in adolescence and adulthood, including multiple avoidance activities (Briere et al., 2010; Cloitre et al., 2009). Specifically, the more types of trauma and neglect experienced in childhood, the greater the number of different problems there tend to be later on, a phenomenon that Cloitre and colleagues suggest may reflect overwhelmed self-regulatory functions.

To the extent that multiple DRBs reflect a more complex trauma history, more need for avoidance, and greater self-regulatory difficulties, the client presenting with multiple DRBs is especially likely to require stabilization and emotional regulation-focused interventions, both early in treatment and thereafter. This suggestion parallels recommendations for extended stabilization in the treatment of BPD (American Psychiatric Association, 2001), which also involves multiple DRBs (American Psychiatric Association, 2013).

Beyond suggesting the need for greater stabilization and emotional regulation, multiple DRBs presents a quandary: Which DRB should be addressed first, or should they all be approached simultaneously? In many cases, the answer revolves around safety: Is one of the DRBs more dangerous or otherwise more problematic than the others? Or is the client involved in several lower-intensity DRBs that are used interchangeably?

As discussed below for high-danger DRBs, when the client is involved in concerning levels of self-injury or triggered suicide attempts, or bingeing–purging to the point of life endangerment, these behaviors should be prioritized, and interventions may sometimes include more extreme measures, such as hospitalization or medication. When DRBs are less immediately threatening, the client and therapist may choose to work out a hierarchy of concern regarding which DRB should be addressed first or to the greatest extent.

In general, unless one DRB appears to be more dangerous than another, the hierarchy of concern approach may be a compromise between focusing on a single DRB and treating all DRBs as equivalent targets for intervention. The hierarchy is formed when the client and therapist create a list of all the client's current DRBs, in order of dangerousness or, if there is no acute danger, relative social or psychological detriment. When one or two DRBs are clearly more concerning, those may receive relatively more attention in treatment than other avoidance responses. When DRBs are ranked as equally concerning, or the difference between (nondangerous) DRBs is small, the clinician and client may choose to work on the etiology of DRBs in general, using general trigger management, emotional regulation skills development, and, perhaps, titrated exposure—including multiple DRB targets on the Triggers-to-Memories Worksheet.

DRB Substitution

It is not unusual to find that when one avoidance behavior is effectively blocked (e.g., though hospitalization, or involvement in a 12-step program that strongly reinforces terminating a specific behavior), but the underlying activation–regulation imbalance has not been addressed, a new avoidance response will emerge. Previously considered evidence of an "addictive personality" (Lang, 1983), new DRBs or substance use, in fact, make perfect sense: They serve a homeostatic, regulating function in the face of overwhelming internal experience and insufficient avoidance. When DRB substitution occurs, the clinician is advised not to pathologize the emergence of a new problem, but instead (1) add this DRB to the RA forms described in this book, (2) determine with the client whether this new DRB requires prioritization, and (3) continue to help the client with emotional regulation skills, trigger management, and emotional processing.

DRBs in the Context of Substance Use

Francis is a 34-year-old truck driver with a long history of "anger issues," which has resulted in several arrests for assault over the years, and, most recently, temporary termination of her parental rights after she hit her 9-year-old son hard enough to leave a bruise. In each of these instances, Francis attributes her behavior to alcoholic "blackouts." She has been compelled to attend therapy, anger management classes, and Alcoholics Anonymous sessions on multiple occasions, but her aggressive outbursts have gone unchanged. Her last therapist noted Francis's childhood history of physical abuse at the hands of her alcoholic father, and her extensive history of binge drinking, which usually occurs before and after aggressive episodes. Her therapist hypothesized that Francis's behavior is triggered by abuse memories and facilitated by the disinhibiting effects of chronic alcohol use.

Similar to the problem of multiple DRBs, it is not uncommon to find that some of those who engage in problematic avoidance behaviors also have substance use problems (e.g., Harned et al., 2006). This makes sense, since both DRBs and substance use may arise from some combination of childhood trauma, attachment disturbance, and emotional dysregulation. Yet, although they share a similar etiology, excessive drug and alcohol use have specific effects that increase the likelihood of DRBs and potentially make them more risky.

The exacerbating effect of substance use rests primarily in its disinhibitory properties. Particularly in the case of reactive suicidality and aggression, compulsive sexual behavior, and self-injury, drug or alcohol intoxication can reduce emotional regulation capacities, intensify triggered emotions, and decrease inhibitions, potentially resulting in more frequent, extreme, and dangerous DRBs. For example, an individual under the influence of alcohol might react to a provocation in a bar with aggressive behaviors that he otherwise would be able to control. Similarly, as is common in ER contexts, an inebriated individual may make an "impulsive" suicide attempt in response to a relational conflict, only to later regret the action and deny suicidality once sober. In such cases, triggering of attachment or trauma memories still occurs, but the extremity of the emotional response, and the behavior used to reduce it, escalate in the context of substance-related disinhibition.

Not only can substance use exacerbate the effects of triggering, but also its anxiety- and arousal-reducing functions may interfere with the client's therapeutic exposure to memories, and thus, the underlying basis for DRBs. Importantly, although a DRB may transiently distract from a triggered memory, it is unlikely to do so during the following treatment session. In contrast, chronic substance use may anesthetize or alter emotional reactivity for considerably longer periods of time. Since problematic substance use often occurs at least on a daily basis, the half-life of most drugs of abuse overlaps with the time during which the affected individual is in a therapy session. In this regard, clinical experience and some research (e.g., Tipps, Raybuck, & Lattal, 2014) suggest that intoxication at the time of treatment can interfere with the activation and processing of memories, thereby reducing the effectiveness of exposure-based interventions. At the same time, however, studies also suggest that therapeutic exposure can reduce posttraumatic symptoms even among those with continuing substance use (e.g., Persson et al., 2017).

In this regard, it is likely that the time period between last substance use and the onset of a treatment session determines whether activation and exposure will be blocked to the point that emotional processing is less helpful. Thus, for example, whereas a client who appears for his appointment in an intoxicated state is unlikely to benefit from RA-based interventions and, in fact, should be gently and nonjudgmentally redirected to home in the safest way possible, another client, whose last substance use was in the prior day, may gain benefit from therapeutic exposure and other interventions as indicated in the literature (Briere & Scott, 2014).

Given these concerns, several suggestions may be made regarding the treatment of individuals who use substances and also engage in DRBs:

- The clinician should be continuously vigilant to safety issues with such clients, since they may be prone to more extreme and frequent DRBs.
- Although it is possible (and often advantageous) to treat substance use and DRBs simultaneously, the greater risk associated with DRBs that chronically occur under the influence of drugs or alcohol may require that substance use be targeted before DRBs, at least early in treatment.
- Therapeutic exposure may be less effective for clients who present for therapy soon after engaging in substance use. Instead, the clinician may choose to focus more on safety issues and less activating

interventions, and reserve emotional processing for later sessions when intoxication is not present.

- Clients who are intoxicated when triggered may have difficulty calling on skills or perspectives they have learned in treatment, including trigger management and emotional regulation techniques. This may mean that, for substance using clients, even more time in therapy should be devoted to teaching and reinforcing these skills, so that they are, in a sense, "overlearned" and thus available even when the client is intoxicated.

- Despite these concerns, the modern clinical literature suggests the benefit of simultaneous treatment of both substance abuse and trauma-related symptoms (Flanagan, Korte, Killeen, & Back, 2016). In the context of RA-based therapy, this means that therapeutic exposure to attachment- and trauma-related memories that underlie DRBs may be appropriate, especially once substance use issues have been at least partially addressed. However, as described in Chapter 8, for those whose emotional regulation capacities are diminished, this work should be done with great attention to the therapeutic window and the principles of titrated exposure.

High-Danger DRBs

Pierre, a 19-year-old man, is currently hospitalized following a near-lethal suicide attempt involving a gunshot wound to the head. Although the bullet glanced off his skull and did not result in immediately identifiable brain damage, this is his fourth serious suicide attempt since age 16, when he drank Drano following a verbal altercation with his mother. His therapist notes that he has never been clinically depressed, although he had symptoms of PTSD and BPD. Instead, all four suicide attempts appear to have been triggered by conflictual interactions with his mother or, in one instance, his older sister. Pierre has a long history of attachment disturbance and trauma, beginning with neglectful and dismissive parenting by his alcoholic mother, sexual abuse by at least two of her boyfriends, and physical abuse and bullying by his older brother, compounded by a general family environment in which both of his siblings, his mother, and Pierre are emotionally abusive and critical of one another.

The obvious greatest danger of DRBs is death or disability. Certain DRBs, especially triggered suicidality and severe binge–purge eating patterns are associated with increased risk of death, but others, such as reactive aggression, compulsive sexual behavior, and self-injury also have contributed to the demise of significant numbers of people. These risks include:

- Successful death-seeking behavior (not only suicide, but also highly risky behaviors; e.g., reckless driving).
- Accidental death (e.g., "low-level" suicidal behavior or self-injury that inadvertently led to death).
- Behaviors that increase the likelihood of violent assaults from others (e.g., reactive aggression, compulsive sexual behavior).
- Life-threatening physical/medical consequences of risky behavior (e.g., electrolyte depletion and cardiac arrhythmias in bulimic purging, HIV infection in compulsive sexual behavior, septicemia in self-injury).
- Danger to others (e.g., aggressive behavior, neglectful parenting, disease transmission).

Life risk may also be present due to other psychological difficulties that are comorbid with DRBs, such as depression, severe PTSD, and psychosis. These disorders or symptoms can lead to suicidality that is not triggered, but, rather, is a response to chronic emotional pain and hopelessness. Psychosis, in particular, tends to exacerbate suicide risk, may impair the individual's capacity to regulate distress and inhibit harmful behaviors, and, by way of delusions and hallucinations, may lead to risky or suicidal behaviors based on misperceptions of reality or internal commands to do dangerous things (DeVylder, Lukens, Link, & Lieberman, 2015).

Given these risks, the first imperative in working with DRB-involved clients is to ensure as much protection from life risk or debility as possible. This is especially true when DRBs involve high potential danger. In this regard, the clinician has two immediate responsibilities: to do whatever is necessary (and possible) to keep the client safe, and to report and warn when the client is a potential danger to others.

Beyond the safety interventions described in this book, higher-risk or debilitating DRBs may also require medical or psychiatric interventions. Although psychiatric medication has not been shown to be broadly helpful in treating complex trauma-related difficulties such as emotional dysregulation, insecure attachment, relational problems, or self-disturbance (Briere & Scott, 2015), it can be useful when comorbidities such as severe anxiety, depression, mania, or psychosis are present. In fact, any client presenting with DRBs who is also experiencing a major depression, severe PTSD, mania or hypomania, psychosis, or serious suicidality should be evaluated for possible medication before the treatments outlined in this book are undertaken. Psychiatric or medical hospitalization also may be warranted when working with high-risk DRBs, the former in the case of potential suicide attempts, severe or disfiguring self-injury, psychosis, mania, or major depression, and the latter when one or more DRBs pose a potential danger of illness or death, for example, electrolyte depletion in bulimic purging. Psychiatric hospitalization is obviously a serious step and may not only result in stigma but also potentially challenge the therapeutic relationship when it is involuntary. Nevertheless, in extreme cases, it may be the only way to maintain safety for the client; thus, it should always be an option.

In a relatively small number of cases, the clinician may also have to protect others from her client. This is inevitably challenging for both client and therapist, because, in contrast to interventions that increase client safety and well-being, intervening when there is danger to others typically involves doing things that are contrary to the client's wishes. Such actions may include notifying police or child welfare authorities that the client poses a threat to the well-being of a child or dependent adult; warning a potential target that the client has made a serious threat; and, when required, notifying authorities that the client is at great risk of spreading potentially deadly diseases such as tuberculosis or HIV. The therapist's exact duty to warn or report danger to others varies by situation and locality, and clinicians should consult an attorney and/or agency protocol to determine what his specific responses to risk should be.

Conclusion

Few would dispute that the brain's capacity to encode the past is one of its most important functions. Without memory, we could not develop culture, transmit knowledge, learn from experience, or navigate our world. At the same time, however, it is hard for the brain to discriminate certain kinds of memories from current perceptions. This is especially true of implicit memory, which, when triggered, provides experiential (e.g., sensory and emotional) information but does not indicate that the input is based in the past. As a result, we can easily make source attribution errors, thinking that we are experiencing the here and now when we are, in fact, remembering the there and then.

This is most problematic when the past was painful or distressing. As described in this book, those with histories of trauma or attachment disturbance are prone to repeatedly reliving the most upsetting moments of their lives as if they are happening currently. This has to be one of the most unfair aspects of life; those who have been hurt the most, through no fault of their own, are often the ones who continue to suffer the most later on. Even more unfortunately, many of the strategies people use to address this kind of suffering ultimately do not work. The behaviors and substances that seem to provide surcease, whether alcohol, methamphetamines, sex, or self-injury, are at best temporary and often sustain or increase distress over the long term.

It is within this difficult situation that the therapist finds herself. Although inevitably tempted to tell the client to "just say no" to the false promise of things that numb or distract, the clinician has a harder task: to help the client engage and address suffering rather than avoid it. This is the *pain paradox* (Briere, 2015): Doing things to stop pain from the past can just drive it underground and make it stronger, whereas allowing

oneself to experience distress can ultimately reduce its intensity and duration. As noted in this book, it makes perfect sense that the client may not
immediately embrace this idea, since much of his life has been devoted to
escaping suffering, not engaging it.

Despite these potential challenges, this book outlines four tasks for
the DRB-involved client:

1. *Through positive relationships, challenge the interpersonal lessons of
abuse and neglect, especially the belief that people are dangerous and relationships are invitations to maltreatment.* This often seems like an antisurvival
proposition to the DRB-involved person: Since people caused much of the
problem, how could they be part of the solution? Yet, as described in previous chapters, a half-century of research indicates that forming a positive
relationship with one's therapist is often the most powerful correlate of
positive clinical outcomes. This is no small task for people who have been
badly hurt by other people.

2. *Learn skills and develop capacities that allow ongoing functioning
despite the effects of trauma and attachment disturbance.* This is not just the
goal of RA-focused therapy, of course. A variety of approaches (e.g., Follette, Palm, & Hall, 2004; Habib et al., 2013; Najavits, 2002; Semple &
Madni, 2015; Wagner & Linehan, 2006) promote emotional regulation
training, which can be one of the most effective single approaches to
adversity-related problem behaviors.

3. *Increase metacognitive awareness of thoughts, feelings, and memories.*
Metacognitive awareness allows the individual to recognize intrusions
from the past as what they are—memories as opposed to current, real-
time events. When fully engaged, this can offer a version of freedom,
since triggered states are, by definition, not "real," and thus ultimately
irrelevant to the present. As noted in Chapter 6, this component is potentially a quite powerful tool in decreasing DRBs, as the client learns to
predict, detect, and manage triggers in the environment that lead to the
activation of distressing memories. It is also challenging for some, however, since it requires that the client see through source attribution errors
and beyond trigger chaining to the "true" nature of reality as it relates to
his triggers and responses.

4. *Process trauma and attachment memories until they are less able to produce negative states.* Some form of emotional processing or therapeutic
exposure is probably present in any effective treatment for adversity-related
distress, whether psychodynamic, interpersonal, or cognitive-behavioral.
Although, as noted earlier, emotional regulation skills development is
often the most immediately helpful approach to trauma- or attachment-
related difficulties, the memories that provide the motive force for DRBs

may also need to be addressed through some sort of exposure and memory processing. Not only does this require therapeutic safety, support, compassion, and sufficient emotional regulation capacities, it may be best accomplished when the pace and focus is under the client's control, not prolonged beyond her tolerance, and interspersed with other, more grounding and relational therapeutic activities.

Ultimately, all of these components reflect an underlying perspective on problematic behavior that emphasizes awareness, acceptance, compassion, and a nonpathologizing view of the human condition. Compassion, in this regard, does not involve pitying the person involved in "bad" or dysfunctional behavior, but rather supports seeing her as someone who innately deserves appreciation, and who is doing the best she can in the face of sometimes extreme suffering. This does not mean that we necessarily give the aggressive, hurtful, or negligent person a "pass," only that we keep in mind the conditions and processes that result in the behavior we want to stop or change. This phenomenological perspective not only discourages harsh or authoritarian treatment, but it also informs the clinician of the operating conditions underlying unwanted behavior, so that suffering can be lessened and behavior can change.

Breathing Exercises

This Appendix contains two breathing exercises. The first, *counting within breaths,* is similar to what Foa and Rothbaum (1998) call *breath retraining.* It teaches the client to breath in a slower, more regular fashion, and can be helpful when he feels nervous, panicky, or triggered.

The second exercise, *counting breaths,* is more meditative, and can be used to achieve deeper relaxation, as well as growing mindfulness. In fact, some version of breath counting is used by many people as a way to achieve a meditative state.

Both of these exercises can be photocopied from the book or downloaded and printed, in a larger size (see the box at the end of the table of contents), then given to the client to use at home. Many clinicians find it helpful for the client to, at least initially, practice one of these exercises at the beginning of each session, with the therapist reading out the instructions in a slow-paced, calming voice, until the client feels that she is able to do it on her own at home.

(continued)

Counting within Breaths

In this exercise, you are learning to slow your breathing down, so that your body and mind can become more calm and relaxed.

- First, sit in a comfortable position. Plan to spend the next 5–10 minutes paying attention just to your breathing. If you are comfortable doing so, try closing your eyes. If you would rather leave your eyes open, that is OK, too.
- Now, begin breathing through your nose. Pay attention to your breath coming in through your nose and into your lungs, then going out. Notice how long each in-breath and out-breath lasts. You don't have to speed up or slow down; just notice what is happening. *Do this for three breath cycles (sets of breathing in and breathing out).*
- Now try to breathe deeper into your body, breathing into and out of your abdomen. Notice that the belly rises with each in-breath and falls with each out-breath. Try filling your abdomen first, then your lungs. And then, when you breathe out, breathe out first from the abdomen, then the lungs. *Do this for three breath cycles (sets of breathing in and breathing out).*
- Now, practice slowing your breath down. Count slowly to 3 with each in-breath, pause, then count to 3 with each out-breath. At the end of the out-breath, pause until you feel the need to inhale again. This should go something like this:
  - *1 (starting to breathe in), 2 (abdomen full), 3 (lungs full) . . . pause . . . 3 (starting to breathe out), 2 (abdomen empty), 3 (lungs empty) . . . pause.*
- Then begin again with **1.** The actual speed of your counting is up you, although it should be slower than usual. Do this for around 5 minutes.

Remember to focus your mind on counting during breathing. If you become distracted by a thought or feeling, or maybe a memory, just wait until the next breath and start counting again. It is normal to lose track of counting. Just start again with the next breath. You are learning to let go of distractions and stay with just breathing. Counting as your breathe in, counting as you breathe out. *1 . . . 2 . . . 3 . . . pause . . . 3 . . . 2 . . . 1 . . . pause. 1 . . . 2 . . . 3 . . . pause,* and so on.

Practice this exercise every day, if you can, either when you need to calm down or just before you go to sleep at night. As you get better at it, you will relax more quickly, because your mind is learning the skill of relaxed, focused breathing.

(continued)

Counting Breaths

In this exercise, you are learning to enter a more deeply relaxed or meditative state. It will teach you how to sit with yourself for a small amount of time each day, and how to focus your attention and awareness on your breath, and only your breath. This exercise tends to increase *mindfulness,* the ability to just be in the present moment, in the here and now: neither thinking about the past or worrying about the future. In this exercise, you can watch your thoughts, feelings, and memories come and go, arise and fall away, as you keep your attention on your breath.

- First, sit in a comfortable position. Plan to spend the next 10 or 15 minutes paying attention just to your breathing. If you are comfortable doing so, try closing your eyes. If you would rather leave your eyes open, that is OK, too.
- Now, take a slow, deep breath, through your nose, hold it for a few seconds, then breathe out. Do that again: Deep breath in, then out. Notice the air move past your nostrils, then into your lungs and belly, then back out.
- When you are ready, start counting your out-breaths. Breathe in, then count **1** as you breathe out. Breathe in, then count **2** as you breathe out. Count each out-breath up to **10,** then start over again, breathing in, then counting **1** as you breathe out again. This should go something like this:
   - *Breathe in, then breathe out while counting 1; breathe in, then breathe out while counting 2; breathe in, then breathe out while counting 3;* and so on, until *breathe in, then breathe out while counting 10.*
- Then start over at:
   - *Breathe in, breathe out while counting 1; breathe in, breathe out while counting 2; breathe in, breathe out while counting 3;* and so on, until *breathe in, breathe out while counting 10,* and then start over at **1.**

That is basically the exercise, sitting quietly, paying attention to your breath, counting each out-breath, until you get to "10," then starting over again. However, the mind being what it is, this is sometimes harder to do than it seems. Instead, what usually happens is that you get distracted by a thought, a feeling, a sound in the environment, an itch, a pain, or wanting to move your body, and you forget what breath number you were on. This is fine. This is a normal part of breath counting, and actually helps you to learn how to return to your breath when you are distracted. When this happens, just notice that you have been distracted and return to counting your breath. Because you have lost track of what number you are counting, just start over at **1.** When you are distracted by things, or feel anxious, it is not uncommon to lose track. Do not be discouraged; this is part of breath training—learning to detect when your mind has wandered away, and then, without judgment, return your attention back to the breath, starting at **1.** You may want to say to yourself at such times, "There is a thought," or "I am having a feeling." Part of the skill you are developing is not pushing those thoughts or feelings away, but, instead, noticing them without judgment, then shifting your attention back to your breath.

With experience, breath counting can be a pleasant part of your day, when you don't have to do anything but be with yourself, counting your breaths, noticing thoughts come and go, and settling into a relaxed state.

Review of Distress Reduction Behaviors (Rev-DRB)

Client name: _____ Date: _____

Behavior	Age first time ever used	Age last time ever used	Number of times in life (estimate)	Used in the last month? Y = yes N = no	Number of times in the last 6 months (estimate)	Number of times in the last week	Number of times in the last 24 hours
Cutting or burning yourself, banging your head, or hurting yourself in some other way, without wanting to commit suicide				Y N			
Attempting suicide because you were upset about something that happened or because of an argument				Y N			
Using sex to calm down or to feel better, or because you couldn't stop yourself				Y N			
Eating more food than you needed, to calm down or to feel better, or because you couldn't stop yourself				Y N			
Gambling to calm down or to feel better, or because you couldn't stop yourself				Y N			

(continued)

184

Review of Distress Reduction Behaviors (Rev-DRB) *(page 2 of 2)*

Behavior	Age first time ever used	Age last time ever used	Number of times in life (estimate)	Used in the last month? Y = yes N = no	Number of times in the last 6 months (estimate)	Number of times in the last week	Number of times in the last 24 hours
Stealing things to calm down or to feel better, or because you couldn't stop yourself				Y N			
Buying things you didn't really want or need, to calm down or to feel better, or because you couldn't stop yourself				Y N			
Physically fighting or hitting someone because you were upset about something that happened or because of an argument				Y N			
Picking at your skin or scabs, or pulling out your hair to calm down or to feel better, or because you couldn't stop yourself				Y N			
Setting fires to calm down or to feel better, or because you couldn't stop yourself				Y N			
Using the Internet to calm down or to feel better, or because you couldn't stop yourself				Y N			
Using pornography to calm down or to feel better, or because you couldn't stop yourself				Y N			

Trigger Review (TR)

Client name: _____ Date: _____

A trigger is something that reminds you of a bad or upsetting thing in your past, and causes you to suddenly feel like you are back when it happened, or to have the emotions or thoughts you had back then. Most people have a few triggers. What are yours?

Someone crying _____

Feeling abandoned or rejected _____

Sexual things _____

Criticism _____

Someone being very angry _____

Someone who is drunk or high _____

Someone raising their hand near you _____

Someone saying mean or abusive things to you _____

People wanting to be too close _____

Family get-togethers _____

Seeing violence on TV, at the movies, or on the Internet _____

Being alone with someone _____

People in authority _____

Competition _____

Being touched _____

Being lied to _____

Someone flirting with you or making sexual statements _____

Someone acting like they are better than you _____

Someone who reminds you of your mother _____

Someone who reminds you of your father _____

Being let down by someone _____

Being yelled at _____

Mean or dirty looks _____

Being laughed at _____

Being accused of something you didn't do _____

Being ignored _____

(continued)

Feeling alone _____

Other triggers: _____   _____   _____

Pick up to three of your worst triggers from above, and answer the questions below:

Trigger #1: _____

What do you _feel_ when you are triggered? (Mark all that pertain.)

Fear or anxiety _____   Anger _____   Sadness _____   Confusion _____

Shame _____   Disgust _____   Guilt _____   Embarrassment _____

Sexual excitement _____   Hunger _____   Alone _____   Emptiness _____

Horror _____   Betrayal _____   Grief _____   Humiliation _____

Of the feelings you chose, which are the worst two? _____   _____

What do you _think_ when you are triggered? (Mark all that pertain.)

You need to escape _____   You are helpless _____   Things are hopeless _____

You want to hurt yourself _____   You want to hurt someone else _____

You hate yourself _____   You hate someone else _____

You have been abandoned _____   You are ugly or disgusting _____

Nobody loves you _____   You are in trouble _____   You are going to die _____

You are a bad person _____   Something bad is about to happen _____

You are in danger _____

Of the thoughts you chose, which are the worst two? _____   _____

What else happens when you are triggered? (Mark all that pertain.)

A flashback _____   You space out or go away in your mind _____   You get a headache _____

Bodily reactions (like rapid heartbeat, shortness of breath, dizziness) _____

Nausea _____   You have to do something to make the feelings go away _____

You faint or pass out _____

You notice that your reaction is too strong or doesn't fit the situation _____

Trigger #2: _____

What do you _feel_ when you are triggered? (Mark all that pertain.)

Fear or anxiety _____   Anger _____   Sadness _____   Confusion _____

Shame _____   Disgust _____   Guilt _____   Embarrassment _____

Sexual excitement _____   Hunger _____   Alone _____   Emptiness _____

Horror _____   Betrayal _____   Grief _____   Humiliation _____

Of the feelings you chose, which are the worst two? _____   _____

(continued)

What do you _think_ when you are triggered? (Mark all that pertain.)

You need to escape _____ You are helpless _____ Things are hopeless _____

You want to hurt yourself _____ You want to hurt someone else _____

You hate yourself _____ You hate someone else _____

You have been abandoned _____ You are ugly or disgusting _____

Nobody loves you _____ You are in trouble _____ You are going to die _____

You are a bad person _____ Something bad is about to happen _____

You are in danger _____

Of the thoughts you chose, which are the worst two? _____ _____

What else happens when you are triggered? (Mark all that pertain.)

A flashback _____ You space out or go away in your mind _____ You get a headache _____

Bodily reactions (like rapid heartbeat, shortness of breath, dizziness) _____

Nausea _____ You have to do something to make the feelings go away _____

You faint or pass out _____

You notice that your reaction is too strong or doesn't fit the situation _____

Trigger #3: _____

What do you _feel_ when you are triggered? (Mark all that pertain.)

Fear or anxiety _____	Anger _____	Sadness _____	Confusion _____
Shame _____	Disgust _____	Guilt _____	Embarrassment _____
Sexual excitement _____	Hunger _____	Alone _____	Emptiness _____
Horror _____	Betrayal _____	Grief _____	Humiliation _____

Of the feelings you chose, which are the worst two? _____ _____

What do you _think_ when you are triggered? (Mark all that pertain.)

You need to escape _____ You are helpless _____ Things are hopeless _____

You want to hurt yourself _____ You want to hurt someone else _____

You hate yourself _____ You hate someone else _____

You have been abandoned _____ You are ugly or disgusting _____

Nobody loves you _____ You are in trouble _____ You are going to die _____

You are a bad person _____ Something bad is about to happen _____

You are in danger _____

Of the thoughts you chose, which are the worst two? _____ _____

(continued)

What else happens when you are triggered? (Mark all that pertain.)

A flashback _____   You space out or go away in your mind _____   You get a headache _____

Bodily reactions (like rapid heartbeat, shortness of breath, dizziness) _____

Nausea _____   You have to do something to make the feelings go away _____

You faint or pass out _____

You notice that your reaction is too strong or doesn't fit the situation _____

Trigger #____: _____

What do you _feel_ when you are triggered? (Mark all that pertain.)

Fear or anxiety _____	Anger _____	Sadness _____	Confusion _____
Shame _____	Disgust _____	Guilt _____	Embarrassment _____
Sexual excitement _____	Hunger _____	Alone _____	Emptiness _____
Horror _____	Betrayal _____	Grief _____	Humiliation _____

Of the feelings you chose, which are the worst two? _____ _____

What do you _think_ when you are triggered? (Mark all that pertain.)

You need to escape _____   You are helpless _____   Things are hopeless _____

You want to hurt yourself _____   You want to hurt someone else _____

You hate yourself _____   You hate someone else _____

You have been abandoned _____   You are ugly or disgusting _____

Nobody loves you _____   You are in trouble _____   You are going to die _____

You are a bad person _____   Something bad is about to happen _____

You are in danger _____

Of the thoughts you chose, which are the worst two? _____ _____

What else happens when you are triggered? (Mark all that pertain.)

A flashback _____   You space out or go away in your mind _____   You get a headache _____

Bodily reactions (like rapid heartbeat, shortness of breath, dizziness) _____

Nausea _____   You have to do something to make the feelings go away _____

You faint or pass out _____

You notice that your reaction is too strong or doesn't fit the situation _____

Functions of Distress Reduction Behaviors (F-DRB)

Client name: _____ Date: _____

From the following list, pick up to three behaviors that you most want to change.

#1. Cutting or burning yourself, banging your head, or hurting yourself in some other way without wanting to commit suicide _____

#2. Attempting suicide because you were upset about something that happened or because of an argument _____

#3. Sexual behavior that got you into trouble or created problems for you _____

#4. Binge eating _____

#5. Gambling that got you into trouble or created problems for you _____

#6. Stealing things that you didn't really need _____

#7. Buying things you didn't really need _____

#8. Physically fighting or hitting someone because you were upset about something that happened _____

#9. Picking at your skin or scabs, or pulling out your hair _____

#10. Setting fires _____

#11. Using the Internet so much that you had problems in relationships, at work, or personally _____

#12. Using pornography so much that you had problems in relationships, at work, or personally _____

Now, indicate the reasons why you use each one.

Behavior (write the # and a brief description): _____

_____

_____

Reasons for behavior

To distract yourself from your problems _____   To stop feeling numb _____

To let people know how you feel _____   To stop memories _____

To block thoughts _____   To stop upsetting feelings _____

To stop a flashback _____   To feel good so you couldn't feel bad _____

To feel important _____   To control others _____

To get the anger out _____   To punish yourself _____

(continued)

To feel back in your body _____   To get even with someone _____

So someone would pay attention to you _____   To soothe yourself _____

To feel connection with someone _____   To stop feeling empty _____

Behavior (write the # and a brief description): _____

_____

_____

Reasons for behavior

To distract yourself from your problems _____   To stop feeling numb _____

To let people know how you feel _____   To stop memories _____

To block thoughts _____   To stop upsetting feelings _____

To stop a flashback _____   To feel good so you couldn't feel bad _____

To feel important _____   To control others _____

To get the anger out _____   To punish yourself _____

To feel back in your body _____   To get even with someone _____

So someone would pay attention to you _____   To soothe yourself _____

To feel connection with someone _____   To stop feeling empty _____

Behavior (write the # and a brief description): _____

_____

_____

Reasons for behavior

To distract yourself from your problems _____   To stop feeling numb _____

To let people know how you feel _____   To stop memories _____

To block thoughts _____   To stop upsetting feelings _____

To stop a flashback _____   To feel good so you couldn't feel bad _____

To feel important _____   To control others _____

To get the anger out _____   To punish yourself _____

To feel back in your body _____   To get even with someone _____

So someone would pay attention to you _____   To soothe yourself _____

To feel connection with someone _____   To stop feeling empty _____

Triggers-to-Memories Worksheet (TMW)

Client name: _____   Date: _____

Place checkmarks next to the 5–10 triggers that make you feel the most upset or that produce the biggest problems for you:

Someone crying ____

Feeling abandoned or rejected ____

Sexual things ____

Criticism ____

Someone being very angry ____

Someone who is drunk or high ____

Someone raising their hand near you ____

Someone saying mean or abusive things to you ____

People wanting to be too close ____

Family get-togethers ____

Seeing violence on TV, at the movies, or on the Internet ____

Being alone with someone ____

People in authority ____

Competition ____

Being touched ____

Being lied to ____

Someone flirting with you or making sexual statements ____

Someone acting like they are better than you ____

Someone who reminds you of your mother ____

Someone who reminds you of your father ____

Being let down by someone ____

Being yelled at ____

Mean or dirty looks ____

Being laughed at ____

Being accused of something you didn't do ____

Being ignored ____

Feeling alone ____

Feeling controlled by someonee ____

Other triggers: _____   _____   _____

(continued)

Triggers-to-Memories Worksheet (TMW) *(page 2 of 2)*

For each of the triggers you chose, try to connect the trigger to a specific upsetting memory or memories of things that happened to you in the past. This may not be possible for some triggers. Just do the best you can.

Trigger	Memory or memories

In-Session Emotional Regulation and Activation Scale (ERAS)

Client name: _____ Date: _____

Estimated Level of Emotional Regulation This Session

1. **Down-regulation capacity in session**	1 Low	2	3	4 High
2. **Distress tolerance in session**	1 Low	2	3	4 High
3. **Tendency to be overwhelmed by activation**	1 High	2	3	4 Low
4. **Metacognitive awareness in session**	1 Low	2	3	4 High
5. **Level of dissociation in session**	1 High	2	3	4 Low
Overall estimate of emotional regulation this session	1 Low	2	3	4 High

Estimated Level of Activation This Session

1. **Triggerability in session**	1 Low	2	3	4 High
2. **Intensity of triggered activation**	1 Low	2	3	4 High
3. **Duration of triggered activation**	1 Short	2	3	4 Extended
4. **Level of activated anger**	1 Low	2	3	4 High
5. **Level of reliving**	1 Low	2	3	4 High
Overall estimate of memory activation this session	1 Low	2	3	4 High

Activation–Regulation Balance This Session

1	2	3	4
Overactivated			Well-regulated

ReGAIN for Triggered States

When you suddenly experience upsetting thoughts, feelings, or memories "out of nowhere" that don't make sense or seem too powerful based on what is going on at the moment:

- **_Re_cognize** that something has happened and that you are probably being triggered. You may notice that your responses are stronger or more intense than make sense, you may recognize a trigger in your environment, or you may have thoughts or feelings that usually happen when you've been triggered before. Remind yourself that you are remembering something upsetting from the past, not experiencing the present.
- **_Ground_** yourself. Look around you, try a relaxation or breathing exercise, say positive and supportive things to yourself, or distract yourself if you need to. Let yourself calm down a bit before the next step, *Allowing.*
- As best you can, **_Allow_** yourself to experience whatever is happening, with self-compassion. This doesn't mean you let yourself be flooded by what you are experiencing, just that you let yourself feel as much as you can without becoming overwhelmed. Although you may not know where these feeling or thoughts are coming from, see if you can feel caring and kindness for yourself that you are being triggered, just as you would feel for someone else if they were experiencing what you are.
- **_Investigate_** how you have been triggered, the source of the trigger, and the source of the suffering.
- See if you can figure out:
  o What is the trigger? Is it something you experienced, saw, smelled, or heard?
  o Where the trigger came from, for example from child abuse, witnessing family violence, feeling neglected or abandoned as a child.
  o Why it is so upsetting (what it is about this trigger that makes it so painful).
- **_Nonidentify_** with triggered thoughts, feelings, and memories. Remind yourself that you are not your thoughts or feelings; You are having them, but they do not determine who you are or what you should do. Things you might say to yourself include:
  o "This is not me; these are triggered reactions."
  o "I don't have to do what my mind is telling me to do."
  o "I am remembering the past. What I am feeling is not real."
  o "I am not what happened to me or how people judge me."
  o "These are just thoughts or feelings. They may not be true."
  o "This is my childhood talking."

References

Akiskal, H. S. (2004). Demystifying borderline personality: The cyclothymic–bipolar II connection. *Acta Psychiatrica Scandinavica, 110,* 401–407.

Alexander, F., & French, T. M. (1946). *Psychoanalytic therapy.* New York: Ronald Press.

American Psychiatric Association. (2000). *Diagnostic and statistical manual of mental disorders* (4th ed., text rev.). Washington, DC: Author.

American Psychiatric Association. (2001). *Practice guideline for the treatment of patients with borderline personality disorder.* Washington, DC: Author.

American Psychiatric Association. (2006). *Practice guideline for the treatment of patients with eating disorders* (3rd ed.). Washington, DC: Author.

American Psychiatric Association. (2013). *Diagnostic and statistical manual of mental disorders* (5th ed.). Arlington, VA: Author.

Amir, N., Stafford, J., Freshman, M. S., & Foa, E. B. (1998). Relationship between trauma narratives and trauma pathology. *Journal of Traumatic Stress, 11,* 385–393.

Andover, M. S., & Morris, B. W. (2014). Expanding and clarifying the role of emotion regulation in nonsuicidal self-injury. *Canadian Journal of Psychiatry, 59,* 569–575.

Andreassen, C., Griffiths, M., Pallesen, S., Bilder, R., Torsheim, T., & Aboujaoude, E. (2015). The Bergen Shopping Addiction Scale: Reliability and validity of a brief screening test. *Frontiers in Psychology, 6,* 1374.

Ansell, E. B., Grilo, C. M., & White, M. A. (2012). Examining the interpersonal model of binge eating and loss of control over eating in women. *International Journal of Eating Disorders, 45,* 43–50.

Arabatzoudis, T., Rehm, I. C., Nedeljkovic, M., & Moulding, R. (2017). Emotion regulation in individuals with and without trichotillomania. *Journal of Obsessive-Compulsive and Related Disorders, 12,* 87–94.

Ardino, V. (2012). Offending behaviour: The role of trauma and PTSD. *European Journal of Psychotraumatology, 3.* [Epub ahead of print]

Ardito, R. B., & Rabellino, D. (2011). Therapeutic alliance and outcome of psychotherapy: Historical excursus, measurements, and prospects for research. *Frontiers in Psychology, 2,* 1–11.

Arreola, S. G., Neilands, T. B., & Díaz, R. (2009). Childhood sexual abuse and the sociocultural context of sexual risk among adult Latino gay and bisexual men. *American Journal of Public Health, 99*(Suppl. 2), S432–S438.

Asarnow, J. R., Porta, G., Spirito, A., Emslie, G., Clarke, G., Wagner, K. D., . . . Brent, D. A. (2011). Suicide attempts and nonsuicidal self-injury in the treatment of resistant depression in adolescents: Findings from the TORDIA study. *Journal of the American Academy of Child and Adolescent Psychiatry, 50,* 772–781.

Azmitia, M. (1992). Expertise, private speech, and the development of self-regulation. In R. M. Diaz & L. E. Berk (Eds.), *Private speech: From social interaction to self-regulation* (pp. 101–122). Hillsdale, NJ: Erlbaum.

Babcock, J. C., Jacobson, N. S., Gottman, J. M., & Yerington, T. P. (2000). Attachment, emotional regulation, and the function of marital violence: Differences between secure, preoccupied, and dismissing violent and nonviolent husbands. *Journal of Family Violence, 15,* 391–409.

Baer, J. C., & Martinez, C. D. (2006). Child maltreatment and insecure attachment: A meta-analysis. *Journal of Reproductive and Infant Psychology, 24,* 187–197.

Baer, R. A. (2003). Mindfulness training as a clinical intervention: A conceptual and empirical review. *Clinical Psychology: Science and Practice, 10,* 125–143.

Baker, A., Mystkowsk, J., Culver, N., Yi, R., Mortazavi, A., & Craske, M. G. (2010). Does habituation matter?: Emotional processing theory and exposure therapy for acrophobia. *Behaviour Research and Therapy, 48,* 1139–1143.

Ball, J. S., & Links, P. S. (2009). Borderline personality disorder and childhood trauma: Evidence for a causal relationship. *Current Psychiatry Reports, 11,* 63–68.

Bartholomew, K., & Horowitz, L. M. (1991). Attachment styles among young adults: A test of a four-category model. *Journal of Personality and Social Psychology, 61,* 226–244.

Bateman, A., & Fonagy, P. (2010). Mentalization-based treatment for borderline personality disorder. *World Psychiatry, 9,* 11–15.

Bauer, P. J., & Fivush, R. (2010). Context and consequences of autobiographical memory development. *Cognitive Development, 25,* 303–308.

Beck, A. T., Kovacs, M., & Weissman, A. (1975). Hopelessness and suicidal behavior: An overview. *Journal of the American Medical Association, 234,* 1146–1149.

Beck, A. T., Kovacs, M., & Weissman, A. (1979). Assessment of suicidal intention: The Scale for Suicide Ideation. *Journal of Consulting and Clinical Psychology, 47,* 343–352.

Becker, E., Rankin, E., & Rickel, A. U. (1998). *High-risk sexual behavior: Intervention with vulnerable populations.* New York: Plenum Press.

Bedics, J. D., Atkins, D. C., Harned, M. S., & Linehan, M. M. (2015). The therapeutic alliance as a predictor of outcome in dialectical behavior therapy versus nonbehavioral psychotherapy by experts for borderline personality disorder. *Psychotherapy (Chicago), 52,* 67–77.

Bernstein, D. P., Stein, J. A., Newcomb, M. D., Walker, E., Pogge, D., Ahluvalia, T., . . . Zule W. (2003). Development and validation of a brief screening version of the Childhood Trauma Questionnaire. *Child Abuse and Neglect, 27,* 169–190.

Bernstein, E. M., & Putnam, F. W. (1986). Development, reliability, and validity of a dissociation scale. *Journal of Nervous and Mental Diseases, 174,* 727–734.

Bigras, N., Daspe, M.-È., Godbout, N., Briere, J., & Sabourin, S. (2017). Cumulative childhood trauma and adult sexual satisfaction: Mediation by affect dysregulation and sexual anxiety in men and women. *Journal of Sex and Marital Therapy, 43,* 377–396.

Bjork, R. A., & Bjork, E. L. (1992). A new theory of disuse and an old theory of stimulus fluctuation. In A. F. Healy, S. M. Kosslyn, & R. M. Shiffrin (Eds.), *From learning processes to cognitive processes: Essays in honor of William K. Estes* (Vol. 2, pp. 35–67). Hillsdale, NJ: Erlbaum.

Black, D. W. (2007). A review of compulsive buying disorder. *World Psychiatry, 6,* 14–18.

Blair, R. J., & Lee, T. M. (2013). The social cognitive neuroscience of aggression, violence, and psychopathy. *Social Neuroscience, 8,* 108–111.

Blanco, C., Alegria, A. A., Petry, N. M., Grant, J. E., Simpson, H., Liu, S.-M., . . . Hasin, D. S. (2010). Prevalence and correlates of fire-setting in the United States: Results from the National Epidemiologic Survey on Alcohol and Related Conditions (NESARC). *Journal of Clinical Psychiatry, 71,* 1218–1225.

Blaustein, M., & Kinniburgh, K. (2010). *Treating traumatic stress in children and adolescents: How to foster resilience through attachment, self-regulation, and competency.* New York: Guilford Press.

Block, J. J. (2008). Issues for DSM-V: Internet addiction. *American Journal of Psychiatry, 165,* 306–307.

Bodell, L. P., Joiner, T. E., & Keel, P. K. (2011). Comorbidity-independent risk for suicidality increases with bulimia nervosa but not with anorexia nervosa. *Journal of Psychiatric Research, 47,* 617–621.

Bohus, M., Dyer, A. S., Priebe, K., Krüger, A., Kleindienst, N., Schmahl, C., . . . Steil, R. (2013). Dialctical behaviour therapy for posttraumatic stress disorder after childhood sexual abuse in patients with and without borderline personality disorder: A randomised controlled trial. *Psychotherapy and Psychosomatics, 82,* 221–233.

Bonanno, G. A. (2004). Loss, trauma, and human resilience: Have we underestimated the human capacity to thrive after extremely aversive events? *American Psychologist, 59,* 20–28.

Bongar, B., & Sullivan, G. R. (2013). *The suicidal patient: Clinical and legal standards of care* (3rd ed.). Washington, DC: American Psychological Association.

Bostwick, J. M., Pabbati, C., Geske, J. R., & McKean, A. J. (2016). Suicide attempt as a risk factor for completed suicide: Even more lethal than we knew. *American Journal of Psychiatry, 173,* 1094–1100.

Bowen, S., Chawla, N., & Marlatt, G. A. (2011). *Mindfulness-based relapse prevention for addictive behaviors: A clinician's guide.* New York: Guilford Press.

Bowlby, J. (1969). *Attachment and loss: Vol. 1. Attachment.* New York: Basic Books.

Bowlby, J. (1973). *Attachment and loss: Vol. 2. Separation.* New York: Basic Books.

Bowlby, J. (1977). The making and breaking of affectional bonds: I. Aetiology and psychopathology in the light of attachment theory (An expanded version of the 50th Maudsley Lecture, delivered before the Royal College of Psychiatrists, November 19, 1976). *British Journal of Psychiatry, 130*(3), 201–210.

Bowlby, J. (1988). *A secure base: Parent–child attachment and healthy human development.* New York: Basic Books.

Brach, T. (2003). *Radical acceptance: Embracing your life with the heart of a Buddha.* New York: Bantam.

Brach, T. (2013). *True refuge: Three gateways to a fearless heart.* New York: Bantam.

Bracken-Minor, K. L., & McDevitt-Murphy, M. E. (2014). Differences in features of non-suicidal self-injury according to borderline personality disorder screening status. *Archives of Suicide Research, 18,* 88–103.

Bremner, J. D., Southwick, S., Brett, E., Fontana, A., Rosenheck, R., & Charney, D. S. (1992). Dissociation and posttraumatic stress disorder in Vietnam combat veterans. *American Journal of Psychiatry, 149,* 328–332.

Brennan, K. A., Clark, C. L., & Shaver, P. R. (1998). Self-report measurement of adult romantic attachment: An integrative overview. In J. A. Simpson & W. S. Rholes (Eds.), *Attachment theory and close relationships* (pp. 46–76). New York: Guilford Press.

Brickman, L. J., Ammerman, B. A., Look, A. E., Berman, M. E., & McCloskey, M. S. (2014). The relationship between non-suicidal self-injury and borderline personality disorder symptoms in a college sample. *Borderline Personality Disorder and Emotion Dysregulation, 1,* 14.

Briere, J. (1989). *Therapy for adults molested as children: Beyond survival.* New York: Springer.

Briere, J. (1992). *Child abuse trauma: Theory and treatment of the lasting effects.* Newbury Park, CA: SAGE.

Briere, J. (1996a). *Therapy for adults molested as children* (2nd ed.). New York: Springer.

Briere, J. (1996b). *Trauma Symptom Checklist for Children (TSCC).* Odessa, FL: Psychological Assessment Resources.

Briere, J. (2000). *Inventory of Altered Self Capacities (IASC).* Odessa, FL: Psychological Assessment Resources.

Briere, J. (2001). *Detailed Assessment of Posttraumatic Stress (DAPS).* Odessa, FL: Psychological Assessment Resources.

Briere, J. (2002a). Treating adult survivors of severe childhood abuse and neglect: Further development of an integrative model. In J. E. B. Myers, L. Berliner, J. Briere, C. T. Hendrix, T. Reid, & C. Jenny (Eds.), *The APSAC handbook on child maltreatment* (2nd ed., pp. 175–202). Newbury Park, CA: SAGE.

Briere, J. (2002b). *Multiscale Dissociation Inventory.* Odessa, FL: Psychological Assessment Resources.

Briere, J. (2004). Integrating HIV/AIDS prevention activities into psychotherapy for child sexual abuse survivors. In L. Koenig, A. O'Leary, L. Doll, & W. Pequenat (Eds.), *From child sexual abuse to adult sexual risk: Trauma, revictimization, and intervention* (pp. 219–232). Washington, DC: American Psychological Association.

Briere, J. (2006). Dissociative symptoms and trauma exposure: Specificity, affect dysregulation, and posttraumatic stress. *Journal of Nervous and Mental Disease, 194,* 78–82.

Briere, J. (2011). *Trauma Symptom Inventory–2 (TSI-2).* Odessa, FL: Psychological Assessment Resources.

Briere, J. (2012). When people do bad things: Evil, suffering, and dependent origination. In A. Bohart, E. Mendelowitz, B. Held, & K. Schneider (Eds.), *Humanity's dark side: Explorations in psychotherapy and beyond* (pp. 141–156). Washington, DC: American Psychological Association.

Briere, J. (2013). Mindfulness, insight, and trauma therapy. In C. K. Germer, R. D. Siegel, & P. R. Fulton (Eds.), *Mindfulness and psychotherapy* (2nd ed., pp. 208–224). New York: Guilford Press.

Briere, J. (2014). Working with trauma: Mindfulness and compassion. In C. K. Germer & R. D. Siegel (Eds.), *Wisdom and compassion in psychotherapy: Deepening mindfulness in clinical practice* (pp. 265–279). New York: Guilford Press.

Briere, J. (2015). Pain and suffering: A synthesis of Buddhist and Western approaches to trauma. In V. Follette, J. Briere, D. Rozelle, J. Hopper, & D. Rome (Eds.), *Mindfulness-oriented interventions for trauma: Integrating contemplative practices* (pp. 11–30). New York: Guilford Press.

Briere, J., Agee, E., & Dietrich, A. (2016). Cumulative trauma and current PTSD status in general population and inmate samples. *Psychological Trauma: Theory, Research, Practice, and Policy, 8,* 439–446.

Briere, J., Dias, C., Semple, C., Godbout, N., & Scott, C. (2017). Acute stress symptoms in seriously injured patients: Precipitating versus cumulative trauma and the role of peritraumatic distress. *Journal of Traumatic Stress.* [Epub ahead of print]

Briere, J., & Eadie, E. (2016). Compensatory self-injury in the general population: Adverse events, posttraumatic stress, and the mediating role of dissociation. *Psychological Trauma: Theory, Research, and Practice, 8,* 618–625.

Briere, J., & Gil, E. (1998). Self-mutilation in clinical and general population samples: Prevalence, correlates, and functions. *American Journal of Orthopsychiatry, 68,* 609–620.

Briere, J., Godbout, N., & Dias, C. (2015). Cumulative trauma, hyperarousal, and suicidality in the general population: A path analysis. *Journal of Trauma and Dissociation, 16,* 153–169.

Briere, J., Godbout, N., & Runtz, M. (2012). The Psychological Maltreatment Review (PMR): Initial reliability and association with insecure attachment in adults. *Journal of Aggression, Maltreatment and Trauma, 21,* 300–320.

Briere, J., & Hodges, M. (2010). Assessing the effects of early and later childhood trauma in adults. In E. Vermetten, R. Lanius, & C. Palin (Eds.), *The impact of early life trauma on health and disease* (pp. 207–217). Cambridge, UK: Cambridge University Press.

Briere, J., Hodges, M., & Godbout, N. (2010). Traumatic stress, affect dysregulation, and dysfunctional avoidance: A structural equation model. *Journal of Traumatic Stress, 23,* 767–774.

Briere, J., & Jordan, C. E. (2004). Violence against women: Outcome complexity and implications for treatment. *Journal of Interpersonal Violence, 19,* 1252–1276.

Briere, J., Kaltman, S., & Green, B. L. (2008). Accumulated childhood trauma and symptom complexity. *Journal of Traumatic Stress, 21,* 223–226

Briere, J., & Lanktree, C. B. (2012). *Treating complex trauma in adolescents and young adults.* Thousand Oaks, CA: SAGE.

Briere, J., & Rickards, S. (2007). Self-awareness, affect regulation, and relatedness: Differential sequels of childhood versus adult victimization experiences. *Journal of Nervous and Mental Disease, 195,* 497–503.

Briere, J., Runtz, M., Eadie, E., Bigras, N., & Godbout, N. (2017). Disengaged parenting: Structural equation modeling with child abuse, insecure attachment, and adult symptomatology. *Child Abuse and Neglect, 67,* 260–270.

Briere, J., Runtz, M., Eadie, E. M., Bigras, N., & Godbout, N. (2018). The Disorganized Response Scale: Construct validity of a potential self-report measure of disorganized attachment. *Psychological Trauma: Theory, Research, Practice, and Policy.* [Epub ahead of print]

Briere, J., & Scott, C. (2007). Assessment of trauma symptoms in eating-disordered populations. *Eating Disorders: The Journal of Treatment and Prevention, 15,* 1–12.

Briere, J., & Scott, C. (2014). *Principles of trauma therapy: A guide to symptoms, evaluation, and treatment* (2nd ed., DSM-5 update). Thousand Oaks, CA: SAGE.

Briere, J., & Scott, C. (2015). Complex trauma in adolescents and adults: Effects and treatment. *Psychiatric Clinics of North America, 38,* 515–527.

Briere, J., Weathers, F. W., & Runtz, M. (2005). Is dissociation a multidimensional construct?: Data from the Multiscale Dissociation Inventory. *Journal of Traumatic Stress, 18,* 221–231.

Briggie, A., & Briggie, C. (2015). Love addiction: What's love got to do with it? In M. S.

Ascher & P. Levounis (Eds.), *The behavioral addictions* (pp. 153–174). Washington, DC: American Psychiatric Press.

Broadhead, W. E., Gehlbach, S. H., deGruy, E. V., & Kaplan, B. H. (1988). The Duke–UNC Functional Social Support Questionnaire: A measurement of social support in family medicine patients. *Medical Care, 26,* 709–723.

Brooks, H., Rushton, K., Walker, S., Lovell, K., & Rogers, A. (2016). Ontological security and connectivity provided by pets: A study in the self-management of the everyday lives of people diagnosed with a long-term mental health condition. *BMC Psychiatry, 16*(1), 409.

Brown, M. Z., Comtois, K. A., & Linehan, M. M. (2002). Reasons for suicide attempts and nonsuicidal self-injury in women with borderline personality disorder. *Journal of Abnormal Psychology, 111,* 198–202.

Bryan, C. J., Rudd, M. D., & Wertenberger, E. (2014). Reasons for suicide attempts in a clinical sample of active duty soldiers. *Journal of Affective Disorders, 144,* 148–152.

Bureau, J., Martin, J., & Lyons-Ruth, K. (2010). Attachment dysregulation as hidden trauma in infancy: Early stress, maternal buffering, and psychiatric morbidity in young adulthood. In R. Lanius, E. Vermetten, & C. Pain (Eds.), *The hidden epidemic: The impact of early life trauma on health and disease* (pp. 48–56). Cambridge, UK: Cambridge University Press.

Buss, A. H., & Warren, W. L. (2000). *The Aggression Questionnaire manual.* Los Angeles: Western Psychological Services.

Butcher, J. N., Dahlstrom, W. G., Graham, J. R., Tellegen, A., & Kaemmer, B. (1989). *Minnesota Multiphasic Personality Inventory (MMPI-2): Manual for administration and scoring.* Minneapolis: University of Minnesota Press.

Butcher, J. N., Graham, J. R., Williams, C. L., & Ben-Porath, Y. S. (1990). *MMPI-2 monograph series: Development and use of the MMPI-2 Content Scales.* Minneapolis: University of Minnesota Press.

Butcher, J. N., Williams, C. L., Graham, J. R., Archer, R., Tellegen, A., Ben-Porath, Y. S., & Kaemmer, B. (1992). *MMPI-A manual for administration, scoring, and interpretation.* Minneapolis: University of Minnesota Press.

Butler, E. A., Lee, T. L., & Gross, J. J. (2007). Emotion regulation and culture: Are the social consequences of emotion suppression culture-specific? *Emotion, 7,* 30–48.

Butler, S. (1989). Foreword. In J. Briere, *Therapy for adults molested as children: Beyond survival* (pp. xi–xiii). New York: Springer.

Byrne, J. H. (2017). *Learning and memory: A comprehensive reference* (2nd ed.). San Diego, CA: Academic Press.

Byun, S., Ruffini, C., Mills, J. E., Douglas, A. C., Niang, M., Stepchenkova, S., . . . Blanton, M. (2009). Internet addiction: Metasynthesis of 1996–2006 quantitative research. *CyberPsychology and Behavior, 12,* 203–207.

Cahill, S. P., Rauch, S. A., Hembree, E. A., & Foa, E. B. (2003). Effect of cognitive-behavioral treatments for PTSD on anger. *Journal of Cognitive Psychotherapy, 17,* 113–131.

Cavanagh, M., Quinn, D., Duncan, D., Graham, T., & Balbuena, L. (2017). Oppositional defiant disorder is better conceptualized as a disorder of emotional regulation. *Journal of Attention Disorders, 21,* 381–389.

Chamberlain, S. R., Menzies, L., Sahakian, B. J., & Fineberg, N. A. (2007). Lifting the veil on trichotillomania. *American Journal of Psychiatry, 164,* 568–574.

Charlton, J. P., & Danforth, I. D. W. (2007). Distinguishing addiction and high engagement in the context of online game playing. *Computers in Human Behavior, 23,* 1531–1548.

Choi-Kain, L. W., Finch, E. F., Jenkins, J. A., Masland, S. R., & Unruh, B. T. (2017). What works in the treatment of borderline personality disorder. *Current Behavioral Neuroscience Reports, 4,* 21–30.

Cisler, J. M., Amstadter, A. B., Begle, A. M., Resnick, H. S., Danielson, C. K., & Saunders, B. E. (2011). PTSD symptoms, potentially traumatic event exposure, and binge drinking: A prospective study with a national sample of adolescents. *Journal of Anxiety Disorders, 25,* 978–987.

Claes, L., Bijttebier, P., Van den Eynde, F., Mitchell, J. E., Faber, R., de Zwaan, M., & Mueller, A. (2010). Emotional reactivity and self-regulation in relation to compulsive buying. *Personality and Individual Differences, 49,* 526–530.

Cloitre, M. (2015). The "one size fits all" approach to trauma treatment: Should we be satisfied? *European Journal of Psychotraumatology, 6.* [Epub ahead of print]

Cloitre, M., Cohen, L. R., & Koenen, K. C. (2006). *Treating survivors of childhood abuse: Psychotherapy for the interrupted life.* New York: Guilford Press.

Cloitre, M., Garvert, D., Weiss, B., Carlson, E., & Bryant, R. (2014). Distinguishing PTSD, complex PTSD, and borderline personality disorder: A latent class analysis. *European Journal of Psychotraumatology, 5.* [Epub ahead of print]

Cloitre, M., Koenen, K. C., Cohen, L. R., & Han, H. (2002). Skills training in affective and interpersonal regulation followed by exposure: A phase-based treatment for PTSD related to childhood abuse. *Journal of Consulting and Clinical Psychology, 70,* 1067–1074.

Cloitre, M., Stolbach, B. C., Herman, J. L., van der Kolk, B., Pynoos, R., Wang, J., & Petkova, E. (2009). A developmental approach to complex PTSD: Childhood and adult cumulative trauma as predictors of symptom complexity. *Journal of Traumatic Stress, 22,* 399–408.

Coelho, H. F., Canter, P. H., & Ernst, E. (2007). Mindfulness-based cognitive therapy: Evaluating current evidence and informing future research. *Journal of Consulting and Clinical Psychology, 75,* 1000–1005.

Connors, R. (1996). Self-injury in trauma survivors: 1. Functions and meanings. *American Journal of Orthopsychiatry, 66,* 197–206.

Courtois, C. A., & Ford, J. D. (2015). *Treatment of complex trauma: A sequenced, relationship-based approach.* New York: Guilford Press.

Courtois, C. A., Ford, J. D., & Cloitre, M. (2009). Best practices in psychotherapy for adults. In C. A. Courtois & J. D. Ford (Eds.), *Treating complex traumatic stress disorders: An evidence based guide.* (pp. 82–103). New York: Guilford Press.

Craske, M. G., Treanor, M., Conway, C., Zbozinek, T., & Vervliet, B. (2014). Maximizing exposure therapy: An inhibitory learning approach. *Behaviour Research and Therapy, 58,* 10–23.

Cronin, E., Brand, B. L., & Mattanah, J. F. (2014). The impact of the therapeutic alliance on treatment outcome in patients with dissociative disorders. *European Journal of Psychotraumatology, 5.* [Epub ahead of print]

Currie, S. R., Hodgins, D. C., & Casey, D. M. (2013). Validity of the Problem Gambling Severity Index interpretive categories. *Journal of Gambling Studies, 29,* 311–327.

Dahl, A. A. (2008). Controversies in diagnosis, classification and treatment of borderline personality disorder. *Current Opinion in Psychiatry, 21,* 78–83.

Dalenberg, C. (2000). *Countertransference and the treatment of trauma.* Washington, DC: American Psychological Association Press.

Dalenberg, C. J., Brand, B. L., Gleaves, D. H., Dorahy, M. J., Loewenstein, R. J., Cardeña, E., . . . Spiegel, D. (2012). Evaluation of the evidence for the trauma and fantasy models of dissociation. *Psychological Bulletin, 138,* 550–588.

Deacon, B. J., Sy, J. T., Lickel, J. J., & Nelson, E. A. (2010). Does the judicious use of safety behaviors improve the efficacy and acceptability of exposure therapy for claustrophobic fear? *Journal of Behavior Therapy and Experimental Psychiatry, 41,* 71–80.

DeGruy, J. (2005). *Post traumatic slave syndrome: America's legacy of enduring injury and healing.* Milwaukie, OR: Uptone Press.

Deliberto, T. L., & Nock, M. K. (2008). Exploratory study of the correlates, onset, and offset of non-suicidal self-injury. *Archives of Suicide Research, 12,* 219–231.

Dell, P. F., & O'Neil, J. A. (Eds.). (2009). *Dissociation and the dissociative disorders: DSM-V and beyond.* New York: Routledge.

Derogatis, L. R. (1983). *SCL-90-R administration, scoring, and procedures manual II for the revised version* (2nd ed.). Towson, MD: Clinical Psychometrics Research.

DeVylder, J. E., Lukens, E. P., Link, B. G., & Lieberman, J. A. (2015). Suicidal ideation and suicide attempts among adults with psychotic experiences: Data from the Collaborative Psychiatric Epidemiology Surveys. *JAMA Psychiatry, 72,* 219–225.

Di Trani, M., Renzi, A., Vari, C., Zavattini, G. C., & Solano, L. (2017). Gambling disorder and affect regulation: The role of alexithymia and attachment style. *Journal of Gambling Studies, 33,* 649–659.

Dodge, K. A. (1991). The structure and function of reactive and proactive aggression. In D. J. Pepler & K. H. Rubin (Eds.), *The development and treatment of childhood aggression* (pp. 201–218). Hillsdale, NJ: Erlbaum.

Dubo, E. D., Zanarini, M. C., Lewis, R. E., & Williams, A. A. (1997). Childhood antecedents of self-destructiveness in borderline personality disorder. *Canadian Journal of Psychiatry, 42,* 63–69.

Duckworth, M. P., & Follette, V. M. (2012). *Retraumatization: Assessment, treatment, and prevention.* New York: Routledge.

Dutton, D. G. (1998). *The abusive personality: Violence and control in intimate relationships.* New York: Guilford Press.

Dutton, M. A. (2015). Mindfulness-based stress reduction for underserved trauma populations. In V. M. Follette, J. Briere, D. Rozelle, J. W. Hopper, & D. I. Rome (Eds.), *Mindfulness-oriented interventions for trauma: Integrating contemplative practices* (pp. 243–256). New York: Guilford Press.

Dvir, Y., Ford, J. D., Hill, M., & Frazier, J. A. (2014). Childhood maltreatment: Emotional dysregulation, and psychiatric comorbidities. *Harvard Review of Psychiatry, 22,* 149–161.

Eichenberg, C., Schott, M., Decker, O., & Sindelar, B. (2017). Attachment style and internet addiction: An online survey. *Journal of Medical Internet Research, 19,* e170.

Elklit, A., & Brink, O. (2004). Acute stress disorder as a predictor of post-traumatic stress disorder in physical assault victims. *Journal of Interpersonal Violence, 19,* 709–726.

Elliott, D. M., & Briere, J. (1995). Posttraumatic stress associated with delayed recall of sexual abuse: A general population study. *Journal of Traumatic Stress, 8,* 629–647.

Elliott, D. M., & Guy, J. D. (1993). Mental health professionals versus non-mental-health professionals: Childhood trauma and adult functioning. *Professional Psychology: Research and Practice, 24,* 83–90.

Elliott, D. M., Mok, D. S., & Briere, J. (2004). Adult sexual assault: Prevalence, symptomatology, and sex differences in the general population. *Journal of Traumatic Stress, 17,* 203–211.

Emerson, D. (2015). *Trauma-sensitive yoga in therapy: Bringing the body into treatment.* New York: Norton.

Fairburn, C. G., & Beglin, S. J. (1994). Assessment of eating disorder psychopathology: Interview or self-report questionnaire? *International Journal of Eating Disorders, 16,* 363–370.

Farley, M. (Ed.). (2003). *Prostitution, trafficking, and traumatic stress.* Binghamton, NY: Haworth.

Favazza, A. R. (2001). *Bodies under siege: Self-mutilation, nonsuicidal self-injury, and body modification in culture and psychiatry.* Baltimore: Johns Hopkins University Press.

Felitti, V. J., Anda, R. F., Nordenberg, D., Williamson, D. F., Spitz, A. M., Edwards, V., . . . Marks, J. S. (1998). Relationship of childhood abuse and household dysfunction to many of the leading causes of death in adults: The Adverse Childhood Experiences (ACE) Study. *American Journal of Preventive Medicine, 14,* 245–258.

Ferrada-Noli, M., Asberg, M., Ormstad, K., Lundin, T., & Sundbom, E. (1998). Suicidal behavior after severe trauma: Part 1. PTSD diagnosis, psychiatric comorbidity, and assessments of suicidal behavior. *Journal of Traumatic Stress, 11,* 103–112.

Fite, P. J., Raine, A., Stouthamer-Loeber, M., Loeber, R., & Pardini, D. A. (2009). Reactive and proactive aggression in adolescent males: Examining differential outcomes 10 years later in early adulthood. *Criminal Justice and Behavior, 37,* 141–157.

Flanagan, J. C., Korte, K. J., Killeen, T. K., & Back, S. E. (2016). Concurrent treatment of substance use and PTSD. *Current Psychiatry Reports, 18,* 70.

Foa, E. B. (1995). *The Posttraumatic Diagnostic Scale (PDS) manual.* Minneapolis, MN: National Computer Systems.

Foa, E. B., Hembree, E. A., Cahill, S. P., Rauch, S. A., Riggs, D. S., Feeny, N. C., & Yadin, E. (2005). Randomized trial of prolonged exposure for posttraumatic stress disorder with and without cognitive restructuring: Outcome at academic and community clinics. *Journal of Consulting and Clinical Psychology, 73,* 953–964.

Foa, E. B., Hembree, E. A., & Rothbaum, B. O. (2007). *Prolonged exposure therapy for PTSD: Emotional processing of traumatic experiences–Therapist guide.* New York: Oxford University Press.

Foa, E. B., Huppert, J. D., & Cahill, S. P. (2006). Emotional processing theory: An update. In B. O. Rothbaum (Ed.), *Pathological anxiety: Emotional processing in etiology and treatment* (pp. 3–24). New York: Guilford Press.

Foa, E. B., & Kozak, M. J. (1986). Emotional processing of fear: Exposure to corrective information. *Psychological Bulletin, 99,* 20–35.

Foa, E. B., & McLean, C. P. (2016). The efficacy of exposure therapy for anxiety-related disorders and its underlying mechanisms: The case of OCD and PTSD. *Annual Review of Clinical Psychology, 12,* 1–28.

Foa, E. B., & Rothbaum, B. O. (1998). *Treating the trauma of rape: Cognitive-behavioral therapy for PTSD.* New York: Guilford Press.

Foa, E. B., Yadin, E., & Lichner, T. K. (2012). *Treatments that work: Exposure and response (ritual) prevention for obsessive-compulsive disorder–Therapist guide* (2nd ed.). New York: Oxford University Press.

Foa, E. B., Zoellner, L. A., Feeny, N. C., Hembree, E. A., & Alvarez-Conrad, J. (2002). Is imaginal exposure related to an exacerbation of symptoms? *Journal of Consulting and Clinical Psychology, 70,* 1022–1028.

Follette, V., Briere, J., Rozelle, D., Hopper, J., & Rome, D. (Eds.). (2015). *Mindfulness-oriented interventions for trauma: Integrating contemplative practices.* New York: Guilford Press.

Follette, V. M., Palm, K. M., & Hall, M. L. R. (2004). Acceptance, mindfulness, and trauma. In S. C. Hayes, V. M. Follette, & M. M. Linehan (Eds.), *Mindfulness and acceptance: Expanding the cognitive-behavioral tradition* (pp. 192–208). New York: Guilford Press.

Fong, T. (2006). Understanding and managing compulsive sexual behaviors. *Psychiatry (Edgmont), 11,* 51–58.

Fontes, L. A. (2005). *Child abuse and culture: Working with diverse families.* New York: Guilford Press.

Ford, J. D., Chapman, J., Connor, D. F., & Cruise, K. R. (2012). Complex trauma and aggression in secure juvenile justice settings. *Criminal Justice and Behavior, 39,* 694–724.

Ford, J. D., & Courtois, C. A. (Eds.). (2013). *Treating complex stress disorders in children and adolescents: Scientific foundations and therapeutic models.* New York: Guilford Press.

Ford, J. D., & Courtois, C. A. (2014). Complex PTSD, affect dysregulation, and borderline personality disorder. *Borderline Personality Disorder and Emotional Dysregulation, 1,* 9.

Ford, J. D., & Gómez, J. M. (2015). The relationship of psychological trauma and dissociative and posttraumatic stress disorders to nonsuicidal self-injury and suicidality: A review. *Journal of Trauma and Dissociation, 16,* 232–271.

Fowler, J. C. (2012). Suicide risk assessment in clinical practice: Pragmatic guidelines for imperfect assessments. *Psychotherapy, 49,* 81–90.

Fraley, R. C., Waller, N. G., & Brennan, K. A. (2000). An item-response theory analysis of self-report measures of adult attachment. *Journal of Personality and Social Psychology, 78,* 350–365.

Freud, S. (1958). The dynamics of transference. In J. Strachey (Ed. and Trans.), *The standard edition of the complete psychological works of Sigmund Freud* (Vol. 12, pp. 97–108). London: Hogarth Press. (Original work published 1912)

Gannon, T. A., Ó Ciardha, C., Doley, R. M., & Alleyne, E. (2012). The multi-trajectory theory of adult firesetting (M-TTAF). *Aggression and Violent Behavior, 17,* 107–121.

Gannon, T. A., & Pina, A. (2010). Firesetting: Psychopathology, theory and treatment. *Aggression and Violent Behavior, 15,* 224–238.

García-Oliva, C., & Piqueras, J. A. (2016). Experimental avoidance and technological addictions in adolescents. *Journal of Behavioral Addictions, 5,* 293–303.

Gay, P. (1989). *Freud: A life for our time.* New York: Anchor-Doubleday.

Gebauer, L., LaBrie, R. A., & Shaffer, H. J. (2010). Optimizing DSM-IV-TR classification accuracy: A brief biosocial screen for detecting current gambling disorders among gamblers in the general household population. *Canadian Journal of Psychiatry, 55,* 82–90.

Gentry, M. (1998). The sexual double standard: The influence of number of relationships and level of sexual activity on judgments of women and men. *Psychology of Women Quarterly, 22,* 505–511.

Germer, C. K. (2005). Teaching mindfulness in therapy. In C. K. Germer, R. D. Siegel, & P. R. Fulton (Eds.), *Mindfulness and psychotherapy.* New York: Guilford Press.

Germer, C. K., & Neff, K. D. (2015). Cultivating self-compassion in trauma survivors. In V. M. Follette, J. Briere, D. Rozelle, J. W. Hopper, D. I. Rome, V. M. Follette, . . . D. I. Rome (Eds.), *Mindfulness-oriented interventions for trauma: Integrating contemplative practices* (pp. 113–129). New York: Guilford Press.

Germer, C. K., & Siegel, R. D. (Eds.). (2014). *Wisdom and compassion in psychotherapy: Deepening mindfulness in clinical practice* (pp. 43–58). New York: Guilford Press.

Gianini, L. M., White, M. A., & Masheb, R. M. (2013). Eating pathology, emotion regulation, and emotional overeating in obese adults with binge eating disorder. *Eating Behaviors, 14,* 309–313.

Gilbert, P. (2010). *Compassion focused therapy: Distinctive features.* London: Routledge.

Glassman, L. H., Weierich, M. R., Hooley, J. M., Deliberto, T. L., & Nock, M. K. (2007). Child maltreatment, non-suicidal self-injury, and the mediating role of self-criticism. *Behaviour Research and Therapy, 45,* 2483–2490.

Godbout, N., Daspe, M.-E., Runtz, M., Cyr, G., & Briere, J. (2018). Childhood maltreatment, attachment, and borderline personality-related symptoms: Gender-specific structural equation models. *Psychological Trauma: Theory, Research, Practice, and Policy.* [Epub ahead of print]

Godbout, N., Vaillancourt-Morel, M.-P., Bigras, N., Briere, J., Hébert, M., Runtz, M., & Sabourin, S. (2017). Intimate partner violence in male survivors of child maltreatment: A meta-analysis. *Trauma, Violence, and Abuse.* [Epub ahead of print]

Goodman, A. (2008). Neurobiology of addiction: An integrative review. *Biochemical Pharmacology, 75,* 266–322.

Gorla, K., & Mathews, M. (2005). Pharmacological treatment of eating disorders. *Psychiatry (Edgmont), 2,* 43–48.

Gormally, J., Black, S., Daston, S., & Rardin, D. (1982). The assessment of binge eating severity among obese persons. *Addictive Behaviors, 7,* 47–55.

Gračanin, A., Bylsma, L., & Vingerhoets, A. J. J. M. (2014). Is crying a self-soothing behavior? *Frontiers in Psychology, 5,* 502.

Grandclerc, S., De Labrouhe, D., Spodenkiewicz, M., Lachal, J., & Moro, M. R. (2016). Relations between nonsuicidal self-injury and suicidal behavior in adolescence: A systematic review. *PLOS ONE, 11*(4), e0153760.

Grant, J. E., & Chamberlain, S. R. (2014). Impulsive action and impulsive choice across substance and behavioral addictions cause or consequence. *Addictive Behaviors, 39,* 1632–1639.

Grant, J. E., & Kim, S. W. (2002). An open label study of naltrexone in the treatment of kleptomania. *Journal of Clinical Psychiatry 63,* 349–356.

Grant, J. E., Kim, S. W., & McCabe, J. (2006). A Structured Clinical Interview for Kleptomania (SCI-K): Preliminary validity and reliability testing. *International Journal of Methods in Psychiatric Research, 15,* 83–94.

Grant, J. E., & Leppink, E. W. (2015). Choosing a treatment for disruptive, impulse-control, and conduct disorders: Limited evidence, no approved drugs to guide treatment. *Current Psychiatry, 14,* 28–36.

Grant, J. E., Potenza, M. N., Weinstein, A., & Gorelick, D. A. (2010). Introduction to behavioral addictions. *American Journal of Drug and Alcohol Abuse, 36,* 233–241.

Gratz, K. L. (2001). Measurement of deliberate self-harm: Preliminary data on the Deliberate Self-Harm Inventory. *Journal of Psychopathology and Behavioral Assessment, 23,* 253–263.

Gratz, K. L., Conrad, S. D., & Roemer, L. (2002). Risk factors for deliberate self-harm among college students. *American Journal of Orthopsychiatry, 72,* 128–140.

Greene, R. L. (2010). *The MMPI-2/MMPI-2-RF: An interpretive manual* (3rd ed.). New York: Pearson.

Greenwald, A. G., & Banaji, M. R. (2017). The implicit revolution: Reconceiving the relation between conscious and unconscious. *American Psychologist, 72,* 861–871.

Grossman, P., Niemann, L., Schmidt, S., & Walach, H. (2004). Mindfulness-based stress reduction and health benefits: A meta-analysis. *Journal of Psychosomatic Research, 57,* 35–43.

Gvion, Y., & Apter, A. (2011). Aggression, impulsivity, and suicide behavior: A review of the literature. *Archives of Suicide Research, 15,* 93–112.

Habib, M., Labruna, V., & Newman, J. (2013). Complex histories and complex presentations: Implementation of a manually-guided group treatment for traumatized adolescents. *Journal of Family Violence, 28,* 717–728.

Harden, K. P., Carlson, M. D., Kretsch, N., Corbin, W. R., & Fromme, K. (2015). Childhood sexual abuse and impulsive personality traits: Mixed evidence for moderation by DRD4 genotype. *Journal of Research in Personality, 55,* 30–40.

Harned, M. S., Najavits, L. M., & Weiss, R. D. (2006). Self-harm and suicidal behavior in women with comorbid PTSD and substance dependence. *American Journal on Addictions, 15,* 392–395.

Harrison, B. E., Son, G. R., Kim, J., & Whall, A. L. (2007). Preserved implicit memory in dementia: A potential model for care. *American Journal of Alzheimer's Disease and Other Dementias, 22,* 286–293.

Hay, P. P., Bacaltchuk, J., Stefano, S., & Kashyap, P. (2009). Psychological treatments for bulimia nervosa and binging. *Cochrane Database of Systematic Reviews, 4,* CD000562.

Hayes, S. C., Luoma, J. B., Bond, F. W., Masuda, A., & Lillis, J. (2006). Acceptance and commitment therapy: Model, processes and outcomes. *Behaviour Research and Therapy, 44,* 1–25.

Hayes, S. C., Strosahl, K. D., & Wilson, K. G. (2012). *Acceptance and commitment therapy: The process and practice of mindful change* (2nd ed.). New York: Guilford Press.

Hayes, S. C., Wilson, K. G., Gifford, E. V., Follette, V. M., & Strosahl, K. (1996). Experiential avoidance and behavioral disorders: A functional dimensional approach to diagnosis and treatment. *Journal of Consulting and Clinical Psychology, 64,* 1152–1168.

Hebb, D. O. (1955). Drives and the C.N.S. (conceptual nervous system). *Psychological Review, 62,* 243–254.

Heilbron, N., Compton, J. S., Daniel, S. S., & Goldston, D. B. (2010). The problematic label of suicide gesture: Alternatives for clinical research and practice. *Professional Psychology: Research and Practice, 41,* 221–227.

Helbig-Lang, S., & Petermann, F. (2010). Tolerate or eliminate?: A systematic review on the effects of safety behavior across anxiety disorders. *Clinical Psychology: Science and Practice, 17,* 218–233.

Hendriks, M. C. P., Rottenberg, J., & Vingerhoets, A. J. J. M. (2007). Can the distress signal and arousal-reduction view be reconciled?: Evidence from the cardiovascular system. *Emotion, 7,* 458–463.

Herman, J. L. (1992a). Complex PTSD: A syndrome in survivors of prolonged and repeated trauma. *Journal of Traumatic Stress, 5,* 377–391.

Herman, J. L. (1992b). *Trauma and recovery: The aftermath of violence–from domestic abuse to political terror.* New York: Basic Books.

Hildyard, K. L., & Wolfe, D. A. (2002). Child neglect: Developmental issues and outcomes. *Child Abuse and Neglect, 26,* 679–695.

Hjelmeland, H., & Knizek, B. (2010). Why we need qualitative research in suicidology. *Suicide and Life-Threatening Behavior, 40,* 74–80.

Hofmann, S. G., Sawyer, A. T., Witt, A. A., & Oh, D. (2010). The effect of mindfulness-based therapy on anxiety and depression: A meta-analytic review. *Journal of Consulting and Clinical Psychology, 78,* 169–183.

Högberg, G., & Hällström, T. (2018). Mood regulation focused CBT based on memory reconsolidation, reduced suicidal ideation and depression in youth in a randomised controlled study. *International Journal of Environmental Research and Public Health,* E921, pii.

Holtgraves, T. (2009). Evaluating the Problem Gambling Severity Index. *Journal of Gambling Studies, 25,* 105–120.

Homma, Y., Wang, N., Saewyc, E., & Kishor, N. (2012). The relationship between sexual abuse and risky sexual behavior among adolescent boys: A meta-analysis. *Journal of Adolescent Health, 51,* 18–24.

Houck, C. D., Hadley, W., Lescano, C. M., Pugatch, D., Brown, L. K., & Project SHIELD Study Group. (2008). Suicide attempt and sexual risk behavior: Relationship among adolescents. *Archives of Suicide Research, 12,* 39–49.

Hoyer, W. D., & MacInnis, D. J. (2007). *Consumer behavior* (4th ed.). Boston: Houghton Mifflin.

Jacoby, R. J., & Abramowitz, J. S. (2016). Inhibitory learning approaches to exposure therapy: A critical review and translation to obsessive–compulsive disorder. *Clinical Psychology Review, 49,* 28–40.

Jentsch, J. D., & Taylor, J. R. (1999). Impulsivity resulting from frontostriatal dysfunction in drug abuse: Implications for the control of behavior by reward-related stimuli. *Psychopharmacology, 146,* 373–390.

Jobes, D. A. (2016). *Managing suicidal risk: A collaborative approach* (2nd ed.). New York: Guilford Press.

Johnson, J. G., Cohen, P., Brown, J., Smailes, E. M., & Bernstein, D. P. (1999). Childhood maltreatment increases risk for personality disorders during early adulthood. *Archives of General Psychiatry, 56,* 600–606.

Kabat-Zinn, J. (1982). An outpatient program in behavioral medicine for chronic pain patients based on the practice of mindfulness meditation: Theoretical considerations and preliminary results. *General Hospital Psychiatry, 4,* 33–47.

Kabat-Zinn, J. (1994). *Wherever you go, there you are: Mindfulness meditation in everyday life.* New York: Hyperion.

Kabat-Zinn, J. (2003). Mindfulness-based stress reduction (MBSR). *Constructivism in the Human Sciences, 8,* 73–107.

Kafka, M. P. (2010). Hypersexual disorder: A proposed diagnosis for DSM-V. *Archives of Sexual Behavior, 39,* 377–400.

Kalichman, S. C., & Rompa, D. (2001). The Sexual Compulsivity Scale: Further development and use with HIV positive persons. *Journal of Personality Assessment, 76,* 379–395.

Kaniasty, K. (2005). Social support and traumatic stress. *PTSD Research Quarterly, 16,* 1–7.

Karam, E. G., Friedman, M. J., Hill, E. D., Kessler, R. C., McLaughlin, K. A., Petukhova, M., . . . Koenen, K. C. (2014). Cumulative traumas and risk thresholds: 12-month PTSD in the World Mental Health (WMH) surveys. *Depression and Anxiety, 31,* 130–142.

Kellett, S., & Bolton, J. (2009). Compulsive buying: A cognitive-behavioural model. *Clinical Psychology and Psychotherapy, 16,* 83–99.

Kelly, T. H., & Bardo, M. T. (2016). Emotion regulation and drug abuse: Implications for prevention and treatment. *Drug and Alcohol Dependence, 163*(Suppl. 1), S1–S2.

Kerig, P. K. (2013). *Psychological trauma and juvenile delinquency: New directions in research and intervention.* New York: Routledge.

Kernberg, O. F. (1975). *Borderline conditions and pathological narcissism.* New York: Jason Aronson.

Keuthen, N. J., O'Sullivan, R. L., Ricciardi, J. N., Shera, D., Savage, C. R., Borgmann,

A. S., . . . Baer, L. (1995). The Massachusetts General Hospital (MGH) Hairpulling Scale: 1. Development and factor analyses. *Psychotherapy and Psychosomatics, 64,* 141–145.

Keuthen, N. J., Wilhelm, S., Deckersbach, T., Engelhard, I. M., Forker, A. E., Baer, L., & Jenike, M. A. (2001). The Skin Picking Scale: Scale construction and psychometric analyses. *Journal of Psychosomatic Research, 50,* 337–341.

Khoury, B., Lecomte, T., Fortin, G., Masse, M., Therien, P., Bouchard, V., . . . Hofmann, S. (2013). Mindfulness-based therapy: A comprehensive meta-analysis. *Clinical Psychology Review, 33,* 763–771.

Kilpatrick, D. G., Edmunds, C., & Seymour, A. (1992). *Rape in America: A report to the nation.* Charleston: National Victim Center and the Crime Victims Research and Treatment Center, Medical University of South Carolina.

Kimbrough, E., Magyari, T., Langenberg, P., Chesney, M. A., & Berman, B. (2010). Mindfulness intervention for child abuse survivors. *Journal of Clinical Psychology, 66,* 17–33.

King, A. P., Block, S. R., Sripada, R. K., Rauch, S., Giardino. N., Favorite, T., . . . Liberzon, I. (2016). Altered default mode network (DMN) resting state functional connectivity following a mindfulness-based exposure therapy for posttraumatic stress disorder (PTSD) in combat veterans of Afghanistan and Iraq. *Depression and Anxiety, 33,* 289–299.

Kirsch, P., Esslinger, C., Chen, Q., Mier, D., Lis, S., Siddhanti, S., . . . Meyer-Lindenberg, A. (2005). Oxytocin modulates neural circuitry for social cognition and fear in humans. *Journal of Neuroscience, 25,* 11489–11493.

Kleinbub, J. R. (2017). State of the art of interpersonal physiology in psychotherapy: A systematic review. *Frontiers in Psychology, 8,* 2053.

Klevens, J., & Ports, K. (2017). Gender inequity associated with increased child physical abuse and neglect: A cross-country analysis of population-based surveys and country-level statistics. *Journal of Family Violence, 32,* 799–806.

Kliem, S., Kröger, C., & Kosfelder, J. (2010). Dialectical behavior therapy for borderline personality disorder: A meta-analysis using mixed-effects modeling. *Journal of Consulting and Clinical Psychology, 78,* 936–951.

Klonsky, E. D. (2007). The functions of deliberate self-injury: A review of the evidence. *Clinical Psychology Review, 27,* 226–239.

Klonsky, E. D. (2011). Non-suicidal self-injury in United States adults: Prevalence, sociodemographics, topography and functions. *Psychological Medicine, 41,* 1981–1986.

Klonsky, E. D., & Glenn, C. R. (2008). Psychosocial risk and protective factors. In M. K. Nixon & N. Heath (Eds.), *Self-injury in youth: The essential guide to assessment and intervention* (pp. 45–58). New York: Routledge.

Koenig, L. J., Doll, L. S., O'Leary, A., & Pequenat, W. (Eds.). (2004). *From child sexual abuse to adult sexual risk: Trauma, revictimization, and intervention.* Washington, DC: American Psychological Association.

Koerner, K. (2011). *Doing dialectical behavior therapy: A practical guide.* New York: Guilford Press.

Korn, D. L. (2009). EMDR and the treatment of complex PTSD: A review. *Journal of EMDR Practice and Research, 3,* 264–278.

Korn, D. L., & Leeds, A. M. (2002). Preliminary evidence of efficacy for EMDR resource development and installation in the stabilization phase of treatment of complex posttraumatic stress disorder. *Journal of Clinical Psychology, 58,* 1465–1487.

Kornfield, J. (1993). *A path with heart: A guide through the perils and promises of spiritual life*. New York: Bantam.

Kosfeld, M., Heinrichs, M., Zak, P. J., Fischbacher, U., & Fehr, E. (2005). Oxytocin increases trust in humans. *Nature, 435,* 673–676.

Koutek, J., Kocourkova, J., & Dudova, I. (2016). Suicidal behavior and self-harm in girls with eating disorders. *Neuropsychiatric Disease and Treatment, 12,* 787–793.

Krahé, B. (2013). *The social psychology of aggression*. London: Psychology Press.

Krebs, C. P., Lindquist, C. H., Warner, T. D., Fisher, B. S., & Martin, S. L. (2007). *The Campus Sexual Assault (CSA) Study, final report*. Washington, DC: U.S. Department of Justice, National Institute of Justice.

Kubany, E. S., Hill, E. E., & Owens, J. A. (2003). Cognitive trauma therapy for battered women with PTSD: Preliminary findings. *Journal of Traumatic Stress, 16,* 81–91.

Kulkarni, J. (2017). Complex PTSD—a better description for borderline personality disorder? *Australasian Psychiatry, 25,* 333–335.

Ladson, D., & Welton, R. (2007). Recognizing and managing erotic and eroticized transferences. *Psychiatry, 4,* 47–50.

Laier, C., & Brand, M. (2017). Mood changes after watching pornography on the Internet are linked to tendencies towards Internet-pornography-viewing disorder. *Addictive Behaviors Reports, 5,* 9–13.

Lane, R., Ryan, L. R., Nadel, L., & Greenberg, L. (2014). Memory reconsolidation, emotional arousal, and the process of change in psychotherapy: New insights from brain science. *Behavioral and Brain Sciences, 38,* e1.

Lang, A. J., Craske, M. G., & Bjork, R. A. (1999). Implications of a new theory of disuse for the treatment of emotional disorders. *Clinical Psychology Science and Practice 6,* 80–94.

Lang, A. R. (1983). Addictive personality: A viable construct? In P. K. Levison, D. R. Gerstein, & D. R. Maloff (Eds.), *Commonalities in substance abuse and habitual behavior* (pp. 157–236). Lanham, MD: Lexington Books.

Lanier, P., Maguire-Jack, K., Walsh, T., Drake, B., & Hubel, G. (2014). Race and ethnic differences in early childhood maltreatment in the United States. *Journal of Developmental and Behavioral Pediatrics, 35,* 419–426.

Lee, C. W., & Cuijpers, P. (2013). A meta-analysis of the contribution of the eye movements in processing emotional memories. *Journal of Behavior Therapy and Experimental Psychiatry, 44,* 231–239.

Lemoult, J., Kircanski, K., Prasad, G., & Gotlib, I. H. (2017). Negative self-referential processing predicts the recurrence of major depressive episodes. *Clinical Psychological Science, 5,* 174–181.

Leshner, A. (1997). Addiction is a brain disease, and it matters. *Science, 278,* 45–47.

Levy, K. N., Johnson, B. N., Clouthier, T. L., Scala, J. W., & Temes, C. M. (2015). An attachment theoretical framework for personality disorders. *Canadian Psychology, 56*(2), 197–207.

Lewin, K. (1935). *A dynamic theory of personality*. New York: McGraw-Hill.

Lewis, K. L., & Grenyer, B. F. (2009). Borderline personality or complex posttraumatic stress disorder?: An update on the controversy. *Harvard Review of Psychiatry, 17,* 322–328.

Lieb, K., Zanarini, M. C., Schmahl, C., Linehan, M. M., & Bohus, M. (2004). Borderline personality disorder. *Lancet, 364,* 453–461.

Lindsay, D. S., & Briere, J. (1997). The controversy regarding recovered memories of childhood sexual abuse: Pitfalls, bridges, and future directions. *Journal of Interpersonal Violence, 12,* 631–647.

Linehan, M. M. (1993). *Cognitive-behavioral treatment of borderline personality disorder.* New York: Guilford Press.

Linehan, M. M. (2014). *DBT skills training manual* (2nd ed.). New York: Guilford Press.

Lloyd, E., Kelley, M. L., & Hope, T. (1997, April). *Self-mutilation in a community sample of adolescents: Descriptive characteristics and provisional prevalence rates.* Paper presented at the annual meeting of the Society for Behavioral Medicine, New Orleans, LA.

Love, T., Laier, C., Brand, M., Hatch, L., & Hajela, R. (2015). Neuroscience of internet pornography addiction: A review and update. *Behavioral Science, 5,* 388–433.

Lu, W., Mueser, K., T., Rosenberg, S., Yanos, P. T., & Mahmoud, N. (2017). Posttraumatic reactions to psychosis: A qualitative analysis. *Frontiers in Psychiatry, 8,* 129.

Lynch, W. C., Everingham, A., Dubitzky, J., Hartman, M., & Kasser, T. J. (2000). Does binge eating play a role in the self-regulation of moods? *Integrative Physiological and Behavioral Science, 35,* 298–313.

Lyons-Ruth, K., Dutra, L., Schuder, M. R., & Bianchi, I. (2006). From infant attachment disorganization to adult dissociation: Relational adaptations or traumatic experiences? *Psychiatric Clinics of North America. 29,* 63–86, viii.

Lyubomirsky, S., Casper, R. C., & Sousa, L. (2001). What triggers abnormal eating in bulimic and nonbulimic women?: The role of dissociative experiences, negative affect, and psychopathology. *Psychology of Women Quarterly, 25,* 223–232.

Maguen, S., Metzler, T. J., Litz, B. T., Seal, K. H., Knight, S. J., & Marmar, C. R. (2009). The impact of killing in war on mental health symptoms and related functioning. *Journal of Traumatic Stress, 22,* 435–443.

Magyari, T. (2015). Teaching mindfulness-based stress reduction and mindfulness to women with complex trauma. In V. M. Follette, J. Briere, D. Rozelle, J. W. Hopper, & D. I. Rome (Eds.), *Mindfulness-oriented interventions for trauma: Integrating contemplative practices* (pp. 140–156). New York: Guilford Press.

Mahler, M. S., Pine, F., & Bergman, A. (1975). *The psychological birth of the human infant: Symbiosis and individuation.* New York: Basic Books.

Main, M., & Morgan, H. (1996). Disorganization and disorientation in infant Strange Situation behavior: Phenotypic resemblance to dissociative states? In L. Michelson & E. W. Ray (Eds.), *Handbook of dissociation: Theoretical, empirical, and clinical perspectives* (pp. 107–138). New York: Plenum Press.

Marikar, S. (2008). Why do stars steal? Retrieved from *http://abcnews.go.com/entertainment/story?id=4490812&page=1.*

Maris, R. W., Berman, A. L., Maltsberger, J. T., & Yufit, R. I. (Eds.). (1992). *Assessment and prediction of suicide.* New York: Guilford Press.

Markowitz, J. C., Petkova, E., Neria, Y., Van Meter, P. E., Zhao, Y., Hembree, E., . . . Marshall, R. D. (2015). Is exposure necessary?: A randomized clinical trial of interpersonal psychotherapy for PTSD. *American Journal of Psychiatry, 172,* 430–440.

Marsella, A. J., Friedman, M. J., Gerrity, E. T., & Scurfield, R. M. (Eds.). (1996). *Ethnocultural aspects of posttraumatic stress disorder.* Washington, DC: American Psychological Association.

Martin, D. J., Garske, J. P., & Davis, M. K. (2000). Relation of the therapeutic alliance with outcome and other variables: A meta-analytic review. *Journal of Consulting and Clinical Psychology, 68,* 438–450.

Masterson, J. F., & Rinsley, D. B. (1975). The borderline syndrome: The role of the mother in the genesis and psychic structure of the borderline personality. *International Journal of Psychoanalysis, 56,* 163–177.

Masuda, A., & Hill, M. L. (2013). Mindfulness as therapy for disordered eating: A systematic review. *Neuropsychiatry, 3,* 433–447.

Mazefsky, C. A., Herrington, J., Siegel, M., Scarpa, A., Maddox, B. B., Scahill, L., & White, S. W. (2013). The role of emotion regulation in autism spectrum disorder. *Journal of the American Academy of Child and Adolescent Psychiatry, 52,* 679–688.

McConnell, A. R., Brown, C. M., Shoda, T. M., Stayton, L. E., & Martin, C. E. (2011). Friends with benefits: On the positive consequences of pet ownership. *Journal of Personality and Social Psychology, 101,* 1239–1252.

Meerkerk, G. J., Van Den Eijnden, R. J. J. M., & Garretsen, H. F. L. (2006). Predicting compulsive internet use: It's all about sex! *CyberPsychology and Behavior, 9,* 95–103.

Meerkerk, G. J., Van Den Eijnden, R. J., Vermulst, A. A., & Garretsen, H. F. (2009). The Compulsive Internet Use Scale (CIUS): Some psychometric properties. *CyberPsychology and Behavior, 12,* 1–6.

Messman, T. L., & Long, P. J. (1996). Child sexual abuse and its relationship to revictimization in adult women: A review. *Clinical Psychology Review, 16,* 397–420.

Messman-Moore, T. L., Walsh, K. L., & DiLillo, D. (2010). Emotion dysregulation and risky sexual behavior in revictimization. *Child Abuse and Neglect, 34,* 967–976.

Metcalfe, J., & Jacobs, W. J. (1998). Emotional memory: The effects of stress on "cool" and "hot" memory systems. In D. L. Medin (Ed.), *The psychology of learning and motivation: Advances in research and theory* (Vol. 38). San Diego, CA: Academic Press.

Meulders, A., Van Daele, T., Volders, S., & Vlaeyen, J. W. S. (2016). The use of safety-seeking behavior in exposure-based treatments for fear and anxiety: Benefit or burden?, A meta-analytic review. *Clinical Psychology Review, 5,* 144–156.

Mikulincer, M., & Shaver, P. R. (2016). *Attachment in adulthood: Structure, dynamics, and change* (2nd ed.). New York: Guilford Press.

Miller, A. L., Rathus, J. H., & Linehan, M. M. (2007). *Dialectical behavior therapy with suicidal adolescents.* New York: Guilford Press.

Miner, M. H., Coleman, E., Center, B. A., Ross, M., & Rosser, B. R. S. (2007). The compulsive sexual behavior inventory: Psychometric properties. *Archives of Sexual Behavior, 36,* 579–587.

Monahan, J. L., Miller, L. C., & Rothspan, S. (1997). Power and intimacy: On the dynamics of risky sex. *Health Communication, 9,* 303–321.

Morey, L. C. (1991). *Personality Assessment Inventory: Professional manual.* Odessa, FL: Psychological Assessment Resources.

Morris, J., & Twaddle, S. (2007). Anorexia nervosa. *British Medical Journal, 334,* 894–898.

Mott, J. M., Mondragon, S., Hundt, N. E., Beason-Smith, M., Grady, R. H., & Teng, E. J. (2014). Characteristics of U.S. veterans who begin and complete prolonged exposure and cognitive processing therapy for PTSD. *Journal of Traumatic Stress, 27,* 265–273.

Murphy, R., Straebler, S., Cooper, Z., & Fairburn, C. G. (2010). Cognitive behavioral therapy for eating disorders. *Psychiatric Clinics of North America, 33,* 611–627.

Murray, C., Waller, G., & Legg, C. (2000). Family dysfunction and bulimic psychopathology: The mediating role of shame. *International Journal of Eating Disorders, 28,* 84–89.

Myers, M. G., Stewart, D. G., & Brown, S. A. (1998). Progression from conduct disorder to antisocial personality disorder following treatment for adolescent substance abuse. *American Journal of Psychiatry, 155,* 479–485.

Nacasch, N., Huppert, J. D., Su, Y. J., Kivity, Y., Dinshtein, Y., Yeh, R., & Foa, E. B. (2015). Are 60-minute prolonged exposure sessions with 20-minute imaginal exposure to traumatic memories sufficient to successfully treat PTSD?: A randomized noninferiority clinical trial. *Behavior Therapy, 46,* 328–341.

Nadel, L., Hupbach, A., Gomez, R., & Newman-Smith, K. (2012). Memory formation, consolidation and transformation. *Neuroscience and Biobehavioral Reviews, 36,* 1640–1645.

Najavits, L. M. (2002). *Seeking Safety: A treatment manual for PTSD and substance abuse.* New York: Guilford Press.

Najavits, L. M. (2013). Creating change: A new past-focused model for PTSD and substance abuse. In P. Ouimette & J. P. Read (Eds.), *Handbook of trauma, PTSD and substance use disorder comorbidity* (pp. 281–303). Washington, DC: American Psychological Association Press.

Najavits, L. M. (2015). The problem of dropout from "gold standard" PTSD therapies. *F1000Prime Reports, 7,* 43.

Najavits, L. M., & Johnson, K. M. (2014). Pilot study of Creating Change: A new past-focused model for PTSD and substance abuse. *American Journal on Addictions, 23,* 415–422.

Netter, P., Hennig, J., & Roed, I. S. (1996). Serotonin and dopamine as mediators of sensation seeking behavior. *Neuropsychobiology, 34,* 155–165.

New, A. S., Triebwasser, J., & Charney, D. S. (2008). The case for shifting borderline personality disorder to Axis I. *Biological Psychiatry, 64,* 653–659.

Newman, S. C., & Thompson, A. H. (2003). A population-based study of the association between pathological gambling and attempted suicide. *Suicide and Life Threatening Behavior, 33,* 80–87.

Nixon, M. K., Cloutier, P. F., & Aggarwal, S. (2002). Affect regulation and addictive aspects of repetitive self-injury in hospitalized adolescents. *Journal of the American Academy of Child and Adolescent Psychiatry, 41,* 1333–1341.

Nock, M. K., Borges, G., Bromet E. J., Cha, C. B., Kessler, R. C., & Lee, S. (2008). Suicide and suicidal behavior. *Epidemiological Reviews, 30,* 133–154.

Norbury, A., Manohar, S., Rogers, R. D., & Husain, M. (2013). Dopamine modulates risk-taking as a function of baseline sensation-seeking trait. *Journal of Neuroscience, 33,* 12982–12986.

Norcross, J. C. (2011). *Psychotherapy relationships that work: Evidence-based responsiveness* (2nd ed.). Oxford, UK: Oxford University Press.

O'Brian, K. M., & Vincent, N. K. (2003). Psychiatric comorbidity in anorexia and bulimia nervosa: Nature, prevalence, and casual relationships. *Clinical Psychology Review, 23,* 57–74.

Ó Ciardha, C., Tyler, N., & Gannon, T. (2016). A practical guide to assessing adult firesetters' fire-specific treatment needs using the Four Factor Fire Scales. *Psychiatry: Interpersonal and Biological Processes, 78,* 293–304.

O'Donohue, W. T., & Fisher, J. E. (2012). The core principles of cognitive behavior therapy. In W. T. O'Donohue & J. E. Fisher, *The core principles of cognitive behavior therapy* (pp. 1–12). Hoboken, NJ: Wiley.

Ogden, P., Minton, K., & Pain, C. (2000). *Trauma and the body.* New York: Norton.

O'Guinn, T. C., & Faber, R. J. (1989). Compulsive buying: A phenomenological exploration. *Journal of Consumer Research, 16,* 147–157.

O'Neill, S., Ferry, F., Murphy, S., Corry, C., Bolton, D., Devine, B., . . . Bunting, B. (2014). Patterns of suicidal ideation and behavior in Northern Ireland and associations with conflict related trauma. *PLOS ONE, 9,* e91532.

Orsillo, S. M., & Batten, S. V. (2005). Acceptance and commitment therapy in the treatment of posttraumatic stress disorder. *Behavior Modification, 29,* 95–129.

Ouimette, P., & Brown, P. J. (2003). *Trauma and substance abuse: Causes, consequences, and treatment of comorbid disorders.* Washington, DC: American Psychological Association.

Ouimette, P., Moos, R. H., & Brown, P. J. (2003). Substance use disorder–posttraumatic stress disorder comorbidity: A survey of treatments and proposed practice guidelines. In P. Ouimette & P. J. Brown (Eds.), *Trauma and substance abuse: Causes, consequences, and treatment of comorbid disorders* (pp. 1–110). Washington, DC: American Psychological Association.

Özten, E., Sayar, G. H., Eryılmaz, G., Kağan, G., Işık S., & Karamustafalıoğlu, O. (2015). The relationship of psychological trauma with trichotillomania and skin picking. *Neuropsychiatric Disease and Treatment, 11,* 1203–1210.

Pachter, L. M., & Coll, C. G. (2009). Racism and child health: A review of the literature and future directions. *Journal of Developmental and Behavioral Pediatrics, 30,* 255–263.

Palumbo, R. V., Marraccini, M. E., Weyandt, L. L., Wilder-Smith, O., McGee, H. A., Liu, S., et al. (2017). Interpersonal autonomic physiology: A systematic review of the literature. *Personality and Social Psychology Review, 21,* 99–141.

Panos, P. T., Jackson, J. W., Hasan, O., Panos, A. (2013). Meta-analysis and systematic review assessing the efficacy of dialectical behavior therapy (DBT). *Research on Social Work Practice, 24,* 213–223.

Paris, J. (2007). The nature of borderline personality disorder: Multiple dimensions, multiple symptoms, but one category. *Journal of Personality Disorders, 21,* 457–473.

Parnell, L. (2013). *Attachment-focused EMDR: Healing relational trauma.* New York: Norton.

Pearlman, L. A. (2003). *Trauma and Attachment Belief Scale.* Los Angeles: Western Psychological Services.

Peck, K. R., Schumacher, J. A., Stasiewicz, P. R., & Coffey, S. F. (2018). Adults with comorbid posttraumatic stress disorder, alcohol use disorder, and opioid use disorder: The effectiveness of modified prolonged exposure. *Journal of Traumatic Stress, 31*(3), 373–382.

Pelcovitz, D., van der Kolk, B. A., Roth, S., Mandel, F., Kaplan, S., & Resick, P. (1997). Development of a criteria set and a Structured Interview for Disorders of Extreme Stress (SIDES). *Journal of Traumatic Stress, 10,* 3–16.

Persson, A., Back, S. E., Killeen, T. K., Brady, K. T., Schwandt, M. L., Heilig, M., & Magnusson, Å. (2017). Concurrent treatment of PTSD and substance use disorders using prolonged exposure (COPE): A pilot study in alcohol-dependent women. *Journal of Addiction Medicine, 11,* 119–125.

Polivy, J., & Herman, C. P. (1993). Etiology of binge eating: Psychological mechanisms. In C. G. Fairburn & G. T. Wilson (Eds.), *Binge eating: Nature, assessment and treatment* (pp. 173–205). New York: Guilford Press.

Prenoveau, J. M., Craske, M. G., Liao, B., Ornitz, E. M. (2013). Human fear conditioning and extinction: Timing is everything . . . or is it? *Biological Psychology, 92,* 59–68.

Rachman, S. (1980). Emotional processing. *Behaviour Research and Therapy, 18,* 51–60.

Ray, A. (2015). *Mindfulness: Living in the moment living in the breath.* Decatur, GA: Inner Light.

Resick, P. A., Nishith, P., & Griffin, M. G. (2008). How well does cognitive-behavioral therapy treat symptoms of complex PTSD? An examination of child sexual abuse survivors within a clinical trial. *CNS Spectrums, 8,* 340–355.

Resick, P. A., & Schnicke, M. K. (1992). Cognitive processing therapy for sexual assault victims. *Journal of Consulting and Clinical Psychology, 60,* 748–756.

Reynolds, W. (1988). *Suicidal Ideation Questionnaire: Professional manual.* Odessa, FL: Psychological Assessment Resources.

Reynolds, W. M. (1991). Psychometric characteristics of the Adult Suicidal Ideation Questionnaire in college students. *Journal of Personality Assessment, 56,* 289–307.

Reznor, T. (1994). Hurt [Recorded by Nine Inch Nails]. *On the downward spiral* [mp3 file]. Los Angeles: Nothing/Interscope.

Roberts, S., O'Connor, K., & Belanger, C. (2013). Emotion regulation and other psychological models for body-focused repetitive behaviors. *Clinical Psychology Review, 33,* 745–762.

Roemer, L., & Borkovec, T. D. (1994). Effects of suppressing thoughts about emotional material. *Journal of Abnormal Psychology, 103,* 467–474.

Rogers, C. R. (1957). The necessary and sufficient conditions of therapeutic personality change. *Journal of Consulting Psychology, 21,* 95–103.

Rogers, P., Watt, A., Gray, N. S., MacCulloch, M., & Gournay, K. (2002). Content of command hallucinations predicts self-harm but not violence in a medium secure unit. *Journal of Forensic Psychiatry, 13,* 251–262.

Rosenbaum, D. L., & White, K. S. (2013). The role of anxiety in binge eating behavior: A critical examination of theory and empirical literature. *Health Psychology Research, 1,* 85–92.

Rushing, J. M., Jones, L. E., & Carney, C. P. (2003). Bulimia nervosa: A primary care review primary care companion. *Journal of Clinical Psychiatry, 5,* 217–224.

Safer, D. L., Telch, C. F., & Agras, W. S. (2001). Dialectical behavior therapy for bulimia nervosa. *American Journal of Psychiatry, 158,* 632–634.

Safer, D. L., Telch, C. F., & Chen, E. Y. (2009). *Dialectical behavior therapy for binge eating and bulimia.* New York: Guilford Press.

Salzberg, S. (2002). *Lovingkindness: The revolutionary art of happiness.* Boston: Shambhala.

Samson, A. C., Wells, W. M., Phillips, J. M., Hardan, A. Y., & Gross, J. J. (2015). Emotion regulation in autism spectrum disorder: Evidence from parent interviews and children's daily diaries. *Journal of Child Psychology and Psychiatry and Allied Disciplines, 56,* 903–913.

Sansone, R. A., Chang, J., Jewell, B., & Rock, R. (2013). Childhood trauma and compulsive buying. *International Journal of Psychiatry in Clinical Practice, 17,* 73–76.

Sar, V., Akyüz, G., & Doğan, O. (2007). Prevalence of dissociative disorders among women in the general population. *Psychiatry Research, 149,* 169–176.

Schalinski, I., Elbert, T., & Schauer, M. (2011). Female dissociative responding to extreme sexual violence in a chronic crisis setting: The case of Eastern Congo. *Journal of Traumatic Stress, 24,* 235–238.

Scherrer, J. F., Xian, H., Kapp, J. M. K., Waterman, B., Shah, K. R., Volberg, R., & Eisen, S. A. (2007). Association between exposure to childhood and lifetime traumatic events and lifetime pathological gambling in a twin cohort. *Journal of Nervous and Mental Disease, 195,* 72–78.

Schindler, A., & Bröning, S. (2015). A review on attachment and adolescent substance abuse: Empirical evidence and implications for prevention and treatment. *Substance Abuse, 36*(3), 304–313.

Schore, A. N. (1994). *Affect regulation and the origin of the self: The neurobiology of emotional development.* New York: Norton.

Schore, A. N. (2000). Attachment and the regulation of the right brain. *Attachment and Human Development, 2,* 23–47.

Schreiber, L. R. N., Grant, J. E., & Odlaug, B. O. (2012). Emotional regulation and impulsivity in young adult gamblers. *Journal of Psychological Research, 46,* 651–658.

Scott, C., Jones, J., & Briere, J. (2014). Psychobiology and psychopharmacology of trauma. In J. Briere & C. Scott (Eds.), *Principles of trauma therapy: A guide to symptoms, evaluation, and treatment* (2nd ed., DSM-5 update, pp. 259–331). Thousand Oaks, CA: SAGE.

Scott, L. N., Kim, Y., Nolf, K. A., Hallquist, M. N., Wright, A. G. C., Stepp, S. D., . . . Pilkonis, P. A. (2013). Preoccupied attachment and emotional dysregulation: Specific aspects of borderline personality disorder or general dimensions of personality pathology? *Journal of Personality Disorders, 27,* 473–495.

Segal, B. M., & Stewart, J. C. (1996). Substance use and abuse in adolescence: An overview. *Child Psychiatry and Human Development, 26,* 193–210.

Segal, Z. V., Williams, J. M. G., & Teasdale, J. D. (2002). *Mindfulness-based cognitive therapy for depression: A new approach to preventing relapse.* New York: Guilford Press.

Seidler, G. H., & Wagner, F. E. (2006). Comparing the efficacy of EMDR and trauma-focused cognitive-behavioral therapy in the treatment of PTSD: A meta-analytic study. *Psychological Medicine, 36,* 1515–1522.

Semple, R. J., & Madni, L. A. (2015). Treating childhood trauma with mindfulness. In V. M. Follette, J. Briere, D. Rozelle, J. W. Hopper, & D. I. Rome (Eds.), *Mindfulness-oriented interventions for trauma treatment: Integrating contemplative practices* (pp. 284–300). New York: Guilford Press.

Shapiro, F. (1991). Eye movement desensitization and reprocessing procedure: From EMD to EMDR: A new treatment model for anxiety and related traumata. *Behavior Therapist, 14,* 133–135.

Shapiro, F. (1998). *EMDR: The breakthrough eye movement therapy for overcoming anxiety, stress, and trauma.* New York: Basic Books.

Shapiro, F. (2017). *Eye movement desensitization and reprocessing (EMDR) therapy: Basic principles, protocols, and procedures* (3rd ed.). New York: Guilford Press.

Sharma, A., & Sacco, P. (2015). Adverse childhood experiences and gambling: Results from a national survey. *Journal of Social Work Practice in the Addictions, 15,* 25–43.

Shawyer, F., Mackinnon, A., Farhall, J., & Copolov, D. (2008). Acting on harmful command hallucinations in psychotic disorders. *Journal of Nervous and Mental Disease, 196,* 390–398.

Siegel, D. J. (2012). *The developing mind: How relationships and the brain interact to shape who we are* (2nd ed.). New York: Guilford Press.

Siegel, D. J., & Solomon, M. (Eds.). (2013). *Healing moments in psychotherapy.* New York: Norton.

Silverman, S. W. (2008). *Love sick: Secrets of a sex addict.* New York: Norton.

Silvern, L. (2011). Multiple types of child maltreatment, posttraumatic stress, dissociative symptoms, and reactive aggression among adolescent criminal offenders. *Journal of Child and Adolescent Trauma, 5,* 88–101.

Simon, R. I., & Hales, R. E. (2012). *The American Psychiatric Publishing textbook of suicide assessment and management.* Washington, DC: American Psychiatric Publishing.

Simpson, J. S., & Rholes, W. S. (1998). Attachment in adulthood. In J. A. Simpson & W. S. Rholes (Eds.), *Attachment theory and close relationships* (pp. 3–21). New York: Guilford Press.

Skinner, B. F. (1953). *Science and human behavior.* New York: Simon & Schuster.

Sloan, D. M., Marx, B. P., Lee, D. J., & Resick, P. A. (2018). A brief exposure-based treatment vs cognitive processing therapy for posttraumatic stress disorder: A randomized noninferiority clinical trial. *JAMA Psychiatry, 75,* 233–239.

Smart Richman, L., & Leary, M. (2009). Reactions to discrimination, stigmatization, ostracism, and other forms of interpersonal rejection: A multimotive model. *Psychological Review, 116,* 365–383.

Smith, N. B., Kouros, C. D., & Meuret, A. E. (2014). The role of trauma symptoms in nonsuicidal self-injury. *Trauma, Violence, and Abuse, 15,* 41–56.

Spencer, B. (2016, April–June). The impact of class and sexuality-based stereotyping on rape blame. *Sexualization, Media, and Society,* pp. 1–8.

Spiegel, D. (2017). Depersonalization/derealization disorder. Retrieved February 10, 2018, from *www.merckmanuals.com/professional/psychiatric-disorders/dissociative-disorders/depersonalization-derealization-disorder.*

Spielberger, D. C. (1999). *STAXI-2: State–Trait Anger Expression Inventory–2, professional manual.* Lutz, FL: Psychological Assessment Resources.

Sroufe, L. A., Egeland, B., Carlson, E., & Collins, W. A. (2005). *The development of the person: The Minnesota Study of Risk and Adaptation from Birth to Adulthood.* New York: Guilford Press.

Steil, R., Dyer, A., Priebe, K., Kleindienst, N., & Bohus, M. (2011). Dialectical behavior therapy for posttraumatic stress disorder related to childhood sexual abuse: A pilot study of an intensive residential treatment program. *Journal of Traumatic Stress, 24,* 102–106.

Stein, D. J., Grant, J. E., Franklin, M. E., Keuthen, N., Lochner, C., Singer, H. S., & Woods, D. W. (2010). Trichotillomania (hair pulling disorder), skin picking disorder, and stereotypic movement disorder: Toward DSM-V. *Depression and Anxiety, 27,* 611–626.

Stern, D. N. (1985). *The interpersonal world of the infant.* New York: Basic Books.

Stewart, S. H., Buffett-Jerrott, S. E., Finley, G. A., Wright, K. D., & Valois Gomez, T. (2006). Effects of midazolam on explicit vs implicit memory in a pediatric surgery setting. *Psychopharmacology (Berlin), 188,* 489–497.

Stice, E. (2002). Risk and maintenance factors for eating pathology: A meta-analytic review. *Psychological Bulletin, 128,* 825–848.

Stone, M. H. (2006). Management of borderline personality disorder: A review of psychotherapeutic approaches. *World Psychiatry, 5,* 15–20.

Stratford, T., Lal, S., & Meara, A. (2012). Neuroanalysis of therapeutic alliance in the symptomatically anxious: The physiological connection revealed between therapist and client. *American Journal of Psychotherapy, 66,* 1–21.

Strathearn, L. (2012). Maternal neglect: Oxytocin, dopamine and the neurobiology of attachment. *Journal of Neuroendocrinology, 23,* 1054–1065.

Tarullo, A. R., & Gunnar, M. R. (2006). Child maltreatment and the developing HPA axis. *Hormones and Behavior, 50,* 632–639.

Tatnell, R., Kelada, L., Hasking, P., & Martin, G. (2014). Longitudinal analysis of adolescent NSSI: The role of intrapersonal and interpersonal factors. *Journal of Abnormal Child Psychology, 42,* 885–896.

Taylor, F., & Bryant, R. A. (2007). The tendency to suppress, inhibiting thoughts, and dream rebound. *Behaviour Research and Therapy, 45,* 163–168.

Teasdale, J. D., Moore, R. G., Hayhurst, H., Pope, M., Williams, S., & Segal, Z. V. (2002). Metacognitive awareness and prevention of relapse in depression: Empirical evidence. *Journal of Consulting and Clinical Psychology, 70,* 275–287.

Tedeshi, R. G., & Calhoun, L. G. (2004). Posttraumatic growth: Conceptual foundations and empirical evidence. *Psychological Inquiry, 15,* 1–18.

ten Have, M., Verheul, R., Kaasenbrood, A., Dorsselaer, S., Tuithof, M., Kleinjan, M., & de Graaf, R. (2016). Prevalence rates of borderline personality disorder symptoms: A study based on the Netherlands Mental Health Survey and Incidence Study–2. *BMC Psychiatry, 16,* 249.

Testa, R., Grandinetti, P., Pascucci, M., Bruschi, A., Parente, P., Pozzi, G., & Janiri, L. (2017). Attachment disorders in alcohol and gambling addicted patients: Preliminary evaluations. *European Psychiatry, 41*(Suppl.), S396.

Theule, J., Germain, S., Cheung, K., Hurl, K., & Markel, C. (2016). Conduct disorder/oppositional defiant disorder and attachment: A meta-analysis. *Journal of Developmental and Life-Course Criminology, 2,* 232–255.

Tipps, M. E., Raybuck, J. D., & Lattal, M. (2014). Substance abuse, memory, and posttraumatic stress disorder. *Neurobiology of Learning and Memory, 112,* 87–100.

Trace, S. E., Baker, J. H., Peñas-Lledó, E., & Bulik, C. M. (2013). The genetics of eating disorders. *Annual Review of Clinical Psychology, 9,* 589–620.

Treanor, M. (2011). The potential impact of mindfulness on exposure and extinction learning in anxiety disorders. *Clinical Psychology Review, 31,* 617–625.

Tronson, N. C., & Taylor, J. R. (2007). Molecular mechanisms of memory reconsolidation. *Nature Reviews Neuroscience, 8,* 262–275.

Tull, M. T., Barrett, H. M., McMillan, E. S., & Roemer, L. (2007). A preliminary investigation of the relationship between emotion regulation difficulties and posttraumatic stress symptoms. *Behavior Therapy, 38,* 303–313.

Turner, B. J., Dixon-Gordon, K. L., Austina, S. B., Rodriguez, M. A., Rosenthal, M. Z., & Chapman. A. L. (2015). Non-suicidal self-injury with and without borderline personality disorder: Differences in self-injury and diagnostic comorbidity. *Psychiatry Research, 230,* 28–35.

Twohig, M. P., & Crosby, J. M. (2010). Acceptance and commitment therapy as a treatment for problematic internet pornography viewing. *Behavior Therapy, 41,* 285–295.

Tyron, W. W. (2005). Possible mechanisms for why desensitization and exposure therapy work. *Clinical Psychology Review, 25,* 67–95.

Vaillancourt-Morel, M.-P., Godbout, N., Labadie, C., Runtz, M., Lussier, Y., & Sabourin, S. (2015). Avoidant and compulsive sexual behaviors in male and female survivors of childhood sexual abuse. *Child Abuse and Neglect, 40,* 48–59.

Vaillancourt-Morel, M.-P., Godbout, N., Sabourin, S., Briere, J., Lussier, Y., & Runtz, M. (2016). Adult sexual outcomes of child sexual abuse vary according to relationship status. *Journal of Marital and Family Therapy, 42,* 341–356.

Valence, G., d'Astous, A., & Fortier, L. (1988). Compulsive buying: Concept and measurement. *Journal of Consumer Policy, 11,* 419–433.

van der Kolk, B. A. (1996). The complexity of adaptation to trauma: Self-regulation, stimulus discrimination, and characterological development. In B. A. van der Kolk, A. C. McFarlane, & L. Weisaeth (Eds.), *Traumatic stress: The effects of overwhelming experience on mind, body, and society.* New York: Guilford Press.

van der Kolk, B. A., Pelcovitz, D., Roth, S., Mandel, F. S., McFarlane, S., & Herman, J. L. (1996). Dissociation, somatization, and affect dysregulation: The complexity of adaption to trauma. *American Journal of Psychiatry, 153*(Suppl. 7), 83–93.

van der Kolk, B. A., Perry, J. C., & Herman, J. L. (1991). Childhood origins of self-destructive behavior. *American Journal of Psychiatry, 148,* 1665–1671.

van der Kolk, B., Spinazzola, J., Blaustein, M., Hopper, J., Hopper, E., Korn, D., . . . Simpson, W. (2007). A randomized clinical trial of EMDR, fluoxetine and pill placebo in the treatment of PTSD: Treatment effects and long-term maintenance. *Journal of Clinical Psychiatry, 68,* 37–46.

van IJzendoorn, M. H. (1995). Adult attachment representations, parental responsiveness, and infant attachment: A meta-analysis on the predictive validity of the Adult Attachment Interview. *Psychological Bulletin, 117,* 387–403.

van Minnen, A., & Foa, E. B. (2006). The effect of imaginal exposure length on outcome of treatment for PTSD. *Journal of Traumatic Stress, 19,* 427–438.

Van Voorhees, E., & Scarpa, A. (2004). The effects of child maltreatment on the hypothalamic–pituitary–adrenal axis. *Trauma, Violence, and Abuse, 5,* 333–352.

Volkow, N. D., & Fowler, J. S. (2000). Addiction, a disease of compulsion and drive: Involvement of the orbitofrontal cortex. *Cerebral Cortex, 10,* 318–325.

Wagner, A. W., & Linehan, M. M. (2006). Applications of dialectical behavior therapy to posttraumatic stress disorder and related problems. In V. M. Follette & J. I. Ruzek (Eds.), *Cognitive-behavioral therapies for trauma* (2nd ed., pp. 117–145). New York: Guilford Press.

Wagner, A. W., Rizvi, S. L., & Harned, M. S. (2007). Applications of dialectical behavior therapy to the treatment of complex trauma-related problems: When one case formulation does not fit all. *Journal of Traumatic Stress, 20,* 391–400.

Walsh, B. W. (2014). *Treating self-injury: A practical guide* (2nd ed.). New York: Guilford Press.

Walsh, B. W., & Rosen, P. M. (1988). *Self-mutilation: Theory, research, and treatment.* New York: Guilford Press.

Walsh, K., Messman-Moore, T., Zerubavel, N., Chandley, R. B., DeNardi, K. A., & Walker, D. P. (2013). Perceived sexual control, sex-related alcohol expectancies and behavior predict substance-related sexual revictimization. *Child Abuse and Neglect, 37,* 353–359.

Wanden-Berghe, R. G., Sanz-Valero, J., & Wanden-Berghe, C. (2011). The application of mindfulness to eating disorders treatment: A systematic review. *Eating Disorders, 19,* 34–48.

Watts, B. V., Shiner, B., Zubkoff, L., Carpenter-Song, E., Ronconi, J. M., & Coldwell, C. M. (2014). Implementation of evidence-based psychotherapies for posttraumatic stress disorder in VA specialty clinics. *Psychiatric Services, 65,* 648–653.

Weathers, F. W., Bovin, M. J., Lee, D. J., Sloan, D. M., Schnurr, P. P., Kaloupek, D. G., . . . Marx, B. P. (2018). The Clinician-Administered PTSD Scale for DSM-5 (CAPS-5): Development and initial psychometric evaluation in military veterans. *Psychological Assessment, 30,* 383–395.

Wegner, D. M. (1994). Ironic processes of mental control. *Psychological Review, 10,* 34–52.

Weinstein, A., Katz, L., Eberhardt, H., Cohen, K., & Lejoyeux, M. (2015). Sexual compulsion: Relationship with sex, attachment, and sexual orientation. *Journal of Behavioral Addictions, 4,* 22–26.

Weisman, J. S., & Rodebaugh, T. L. (2018). Exposure therapy augmentation: A review and extension of techniques informed by an inhibitory learning approach. *Clinical Psychology Review, 59,* 41–51.

Weiss, B., Garvert, D. W., & Cloitre, M. (2015). PTSD and trauma-related difficulties in sexual minority women: The impact of perceived social support. *Journal of Traumatic Stress, 28,* 563–571.

Weissman, M. M., Markowitz, J. C., & Klerman, G. L. (2000). *Comprehensive guide to interpersonal psychotherapy.* New York: Basic Books.

White, A. M. (2003). What happened?: Alcohol, memory blackouts, and the brain. *Alcohol Research and Health, 27,* 186–196.

White, J. W., Koss, M. P., & Kazdin, A. E. (Eds.). (2011). *Violence against women and children* (Vols. 1–2). Washington, DC: American Psychological Association.

Whitlock, J., Eckenrode, J., & Silverman, D. (2006). Self-injurious behaviors in a college population. *Pediatrics 117,* 1939–1948.

Widom, C. S., Czaja, S. J., & Dutton, M. A. (2008). Childhood victimization and lifetime revictimization. *Child Abuse and Neglect, 32,* 785–796.

Williams, A. D., & Grisham, J. R. (2012). Impulsivity, emotion regulation, and mindful attentional focus in compulsive buying. *Cognitive Therapy and Research, 36,* 451–457.

Williams, A. D., Grisham, J. R., Erskine, A., & Cassedy, E. (2012). Deficits in emotion regulation associated with pathological gambling. *British Journal of Clinical Psychology, 51,* 223–238.

Wolpe, J. (1969). *The practice of behavior therapy.* New York: Pergamon Press.

Wood, R. T. A., & Griffiths, M. D. (2007). A qualitative investigation of problem gambling as an escape-based coping strategy. *Psychology and Psychotherapy: Theory, Research, and Practice, 80,* 107–125.

Wood, R. T. A., Gupta, R., Derevensky, J., & Griffiths, M. D. (2004). Video game playing and gambling in adolescents: Common risk factors. *Journal of Child and Adolescent Substance Abuse, 14,* 77–100.

Workman, L., & Paper, D. (2010). Compulsive buying: A theoretical framework. *Journal of Business Inquiry, 9,* 89–126.

World Health Organization. (2016). Print Versions for the ICD-11 Beta Draft (Mortality and Morbidity Statistics). Retrieved May 23, 2017, from *http://apps.who.int/classifications/icd11/browse/l-m/en/Printables.*

Yaratan, H., & Yucesoylu, R. (2010). Self-esteem, self-concept, self-talk and significant others' statements in fifth grade students: Differences according to gender and school type. *Procedia–Social and Behavioral Sciences, 2,* 3506–3518.

Yates, T. M. (2004). The developmental psychopathology of self-injurious behavior: Compensatory regulation in posttraumatic adaptation. *Clinical Psychology Review, 24,* 35–74.

Yi, S., & Kanetkar, V. (2011). Coping with guilt and shame after gambling loss. *Journal of Gambling Studies, 27,* 371–387.

Yildiz, M. A. (2017). Emotion regulation strategies as predictors of internet addiction and smartphone addiction in adolescents. *Journal of Educational Sciences and Psychology, 7,* 66–78.

Yoon, I. S., Houang, S. T., Hirshfield, S., & Downing, M. J. (2016). Compulsive sexual behavior and HIV/STI risk: A review of the current literature. *Current Addiction Reports, 3,* 387–399.

Young, K. S. (1998). Internet addiction: The emergence of a new clinical disorder. *CyberPsychology and Behavior, 1,* 237–244.

Zachrisson, H., & Skårderud, F. (2010). Feelings of insecurity: Review of attachment and eating disorders. *European Eating Disorders Review, 18,* 97–106.

Zanarini, M. C., Weingeroff, J. L., Frankenburg, F. R., & Fitzmaurice, G. M. (2015).

Development of the self-report version of the Zanarini Rating Scale for Borderline Personality Disorder. *Personality and Mental Health, 9,* 243–249.

Zanarini, M. C., Williams, A. A., Lewis, R. E., Reich, R. B., Vera, S. C., Marino, M. F., . . . Frankenburg, F. R. (1997). Reported pathological childhood experiences associated with the development of borderline personality disorder. *American Journal of Psychiatry, 154,* 1101–1106.

Zayfert, C., & Black, C. (2000). Implementation of empirically supported treatment for PTSD: Obstacles and innovations. *Behavior Therapy, 23,* 161–168.

Zayfert, C., DeViva, J. C., Becker, C. B., Pike, J. L., Gillock, K. L., & Hayes, S. A. (2005). Exposure utilization and completion of cognitive behavioral therapy for PTSD in a "real world" clinical practice. *Journal of Traumatic Stress, 18,* 637–645.

Zeidner, M., & Endler, N. (Eds.). (1996). *Handbook of coping: Theory, research, applications.* New York: Wiley.

Zeigarnik, B. (1927). Das behalten erledigter und unerledigter handlungen [On finished and unfinished tasks]. *Psychologische Forschung, 9,* 1–85.

Zetterqvist, M. (2015). The DSM-5 diagnosis of nonsuicidal self-injury disorder: A review of the empirical literature. *Child and Adolescent Psychiatry and Mental Health, 9,* 31.

Zimet, G. D., Dahlem, N. W., Zimet, S. G., & Farley, G. K. (1988). The Multidimensional Scale of Perceived Social Support. *Journal of Personality Assessment, 52,* 30–41.

Zimmerman, M., & Mattia, J. (1999). Psychiatric diagnosis in clinical practice: Is comorbidity being missed? *Comprehensive Psychiatry, 40,* 182–191.

Zlotnick, C., Johnson, J., Kohn, R., Vicente, B., Rioseco, P., & Saldiviad, S. (2008). Childhood trauma, trauma in adulthood, and psychiatric diagnoses results from a community sample. *Comprehensive Psychiatry, 49,* 163–169.

Zlotnick, C., Mattia, J. I., & Zimmerman, M. (1999). Clinical correlates of self-mutilation in a sample of general psychiatric patients. *Journal of Nervous and Mental Disease, 187,* 296–301.

Zlotnick, C., Mattia, J. I., & Zimmerman, M. (2001). The relationship between posttraumatic stress disorder, childhood trauma and alexithymia in an outpatient sample. *Journal of Traumatic Stress, 14,* 177–188.

Zoellner, L. A., Feeny, N. C., Bittinger, J. N., Bedard-Gilligan, M. A., Slagle, D. M., Post, L. M., & Chen, J. A. (2011). Teaching trauma-focused exposure therapy for PTSD: Critical clinical lessons for novice exposure therapists. *Psychological Trauma, 3,* 300–308.

Zouk, H., Tousignant, M., Seguin, M., Lesage, A., & Turecki, G. (2006). Characterization of impulsivity in suicide completers: Clinical, behavioral and psychosocial dimensions. *Journal of Affective Disorders, 92,* 195–204.

Zuchner, S., Cuccaro, M. L., Tran-Viet, K. N., Cope, H., Krishnan, R. R., Pericak-Vance, M. A., . . . Ashley-Koch, A. (2006). SLITRK1 mutations in trichotillomania. *Molecular Psychiatry, 11,* 887–889.

Index

Note. *f* following a page number indicates a figure.

223